Christopher Schilling

Analysis of Atrial Electrograms

Vol. 17
Karlsruhe Transactions on Biomedical Engineering

Editor:
Karlsruhe Institute of Technology (KIT)
Institute of Biomedical Engineering

Eine Übersicht über alle bisher in dieser Schriftenreihe erschienenen Bände finden Sie am Ende des Buchs.

Analysis of Atrial Electrograms

by
Christopher Schilling

KIT Scientific Publishing

Dissertation, Karlsruher Institut für Technologie (KIT)
Fakultät für Elektrotechnik und Informationstechnik, 2012

Impressum

Karlsruher Institut für Technologie (KIT)
KIT Scientific Publishing
Straße am Forum 2
D-76131 Karlsruhe
www.ksp.kit.edu

KIT – Universität des Landes Baden-Württemberg und
nationales Forschungszentrum in der Helmholtz-Gemeinschaft

KIT Scientific Publishing 2012
Print on Demand

ISSN 1864-5933
ISBN 978-3-86644-894-0

Analysis of Atrial Electrograms

Zur Erlangung des akademischen Grades eines

DOKTOR-INGENIEURS

von der Fakultät für
Elektrotechnik und Informationstechnik
des Karlsruher Instituts für Technologie (KIT)

genehmigte

DISSERTATION

von

Dipl.-Ing. Christopher Schilling
geb. in Hanau

Tag der mündlichen Prüfung: 22. Mai 2012
Referent: Prof. Dr. rer. nat. Olaf Dössel
Korreferent: Prof. Dr. med. Claus Schmitt

Danksagung

Diese Arbeit entstand im Rahmen meiner Tätigkeit als wissenschaftlicher Mitarbeiter am Institut für Biomedizinische Technik des Karlsruher Instituts für Technologie. Bei der Entstehung dieser Arbeit habe ich wertvolle Unterstützung erhalten, für die ich mich herzlich bedanke.

An erster Stelle gilt mein Dank Prof. Dr. rer. nat. Olaf Dössel für die Möglichkeit, in seiner Arbeitsgruppe an diesem interessanten Thema zu arbeiten, für seine Betreuung, das Korrekturlesen und die Übernahme des Hauptreferates. Sein großes Interesse an dieser Arbeit, seine stete Bereitschaft zu fachlichen Diskussionen und seine hilfreichen Anregungen habe ich sehr geschätzt.
Herzlicher Dank gilt auch Prof. Dr. med. Claus Schmitt, der dieses Projekt initiiert und durch seine Ideen, seine Anregungen und seine konstruktive Kritik bereichert hat und der letztlich auch das Korreferat übernommen hat.

Dr. med. Armin Luik danke ich für die anregenden und gewinnbringenden Diskussionen, den klinischen Input und das unkomplizierte Zusammenarbeiten als klinischer Mitstreiter an diesem Projekt.
Weiterhin gilt mein Dank Matthias Keller für die gute Zusammenarbeit in der Analyse und Klassifizierung klinischer Messdaten, erst als Diplomand und später als Kollege, und für das Korrekturlesen der Dissertation und Martin Krüger für kurzweilige Diskussionen, die freundschaftliche Atmosphäre und das Korrekturlesen der Dissertation.

Bedanken möchte ich mich auch bei allen Kollegen und Mitarbeitern am IBT für die schöne Atmosphäre am Institut und für Ihre Unterstützung bei allen möglichen Dingen, dem EPU-Team des Städtischen Klinikums Karlsruhe, das trotz Klinikstress immer hilfreich und unkompliziert war und auch bei allen Diplomanden, Studienarbeitern und Studierenden, die zu dieser Arbeit beigetragen haben. Im besonderen sind dies Marc Aubreville, Minh P. Nguyen, Stefan Ponto und Bastian Glauner.

Ein herzlicher Dank gilt meinen Eltern und meinem Bruder, die in jeglicher Hinsicht die Grundsteine für meinen Weg gelegt haben und die alle auf ihre Weise zum Gelingen dieser Arbeit beigetragen haben.
Und schließlich meiner Lebensgefährtin Beatrice, die mich stets unterstützt und motiviert hat. Danke, dass Du immer für mich da warst.

Contents

1 Introduction 1
1.1 Motivation 1
1.2 Aims of the Thesis 2
1.3 Structure of the Thesis 3

Part I Basic Foundations

2 Medical Background 7
2.1 Anatomy and Physiology of the Heart 7
2.2 Electrophysiological Basics 8
2.3 The Atria & Atrial Arrhythmias 13
2.3.1 Atrial Flutter 14
2.3.2 Atrial Fibrillation 15
2.4 Catheter Ablation of Atrial Fibrillation 20
2.4.1 Catheter Ablation 20
2.4.2 Mapping 22
2.5 Cell Modeling 24
2.5.1 Hodgkin-Huxley Model 24
2.5.2 Courtemanche-Ramirez-Nattel Model 26
2.6 Bidomain Model 27

3 Mathematical & Signal Processing Fundamentals 31
3.1 Statistic Measures 31
3.1.1 Expectation Value 31
3.1.2 Central Moments 32
3.1.3 Covariance and Correlation 33
3.1.4 Normal Distribution 33
3.1.5 Boxplot 34
3.2 Kernel Density Estimation 34
3.3 Entropy 37

3.4 Analytic Signal & Hilbert Transformation 37
3.5 Fourier Transform 38
3.5.1 Continuous Fourier Transform 38
3.5.2 Discrete Fourier Transform and Fast Fourier Transform 39
3.5.3 Short Time Fourier Transform 39
3.6 Wavelet Transformation 41
3.6.1 Discrete Wavelet Transformation 42
3.7 Principle Component Analysis 44
3.8 Decision Trees 45
3.8.1 Tree Induction 47
3.8.2 Splitting Criteria 47
3.8.3 Optimizing a Tree 49
3.8.4 Class Membership of Leaf Nodes 52

Part II Quantitative Analysis of Atrial Electrograms

4 Introduction and Preprocessing of Atrial Electrograms 57
4.1 Intra-atrial Electrograms 57
4.2 Complex Fractionated Atrial Electrograms (CFAEs) 58
4.2.1 CFAE Classes in Case of Persistent AF 59
4.3 Setting up Databases of Atrial Signals 60
4.3.1 Database of CFAEs 60
4.3.2 Database of CFAEmean Maps 62
4.3.3 Database of Contact & Non-Contact Signals 62
4.4 Preprocessing Atrial Electrograms 63
4.4.1 Baseline Wander Removal 64
4.4.2 High Frequency Noise Reduction 64

5 PCA-based Ventricular Far Field Cancellation 67
5.1 The Ventricular Far Field 67
5.2 Multi-channel PCA-based VFF Reduction 69
5.2.1 R-Peak Detection & Segmentation 71
5.2.2 VFF Removal 72
5.3 Evaluation Method 75
5.4 Results of Ventricular Far Field Cancellation 78

6 Segmenting Atrial Electrograms 83
6.1 Energy of a Harmonic Oscillation 83
6.2 Non-Linear Energy Operator 84
6.2.1 NLEO of an Exponentially Damped Sinus Signal 86
6.2.2 NLEO of a Chirp Signal 86

6.2.3 NLEO of Superimposed Sinus Functions ... 89
6.3 NLEO-based Segmentation of CFAEs ... 89
6.4 Results of CFAE Segmentation ... 92

7 Describing Atrial Electrograms ... 97
7.1 Test and Evaluation of Descriptors ... 97
7.2 Amplitude Statistics-based Descriptors ... 98
7.3 Time Domain Descriptors Based on NLEO ... 100
7.4 Similarity of Active Segments ... 101
7.5 Frequency Analysis of CFAEs, Periodicity Detection ... 103
7.5.1 CFAEmean ... 103
7.5.2 Dominant Frequency ... 105
7.5.3 Characteristic Frequencies ... 106
7.5.4 Power Density Spectrum-based Descriptors ... 111
7.6 PCA-based Descriptors ... 113
7.7 Wavelet-based Descriptors ... 114
7.8 Phase Space-based Descriptors ... 116
7.9 Results of Descriptors for EGMs ... 119

8 Fuzzy Decision Tree to Classify CFAEs ... 121
8.1 Building the Fuzzy Decision Tree ... 121
8.2 Pruning the Tree ... 125
8.3 Validation and Comparison ... 126
8.4 Results of Evaluation ... 127
8.5 Results of CFAE Classification ... 128
8.5.1 Descriptor Results ... 128
8.5.2 Classification Results ... 132

9 Contact vs. Non-contact Electrograms ... 137
9.1 Simulation of Intracardiac Electrograms ... 139
9.2 Detecting Signals with Endocardium Contact ... 141
9.3 Results of Analyzing the Endocardium Contact of Catheter ... 142
9.3.1 Simulated EGMs Results ... 142
9.3.2 Decision Tree Results ... 146

10 3D Visualization ... 151
10.1 Visualization of Atrial Geometry ... 151
10.2 Spatial Analysis — Visualization of Descriptors ... 152

Part III Clinical Applications & Trials

11 Analysis of Coronary Sinus Signals ... 157

11.1 Segmenting & Clustering ... 157
11.2 Results of Coronary Sinus Analysis ... 158

12 Analyzing the Influence of Pulmonary Vein Isolation ... 165
12.1 Clinical Issue & Method ... 165
12.2 Results of the Influence of PVI ... 165

13 Continuous Activity with High Fractionation during AF ... 169
13.1 Clinical Issue & Method ... 169
13.2 Results of Characterizing Continuous Activity ... 170

14 Conclusion ... 175

Part IV Appendix

A Boxplots of all Introduced Descriptors ... 181
A.1 CFAE Class Descriptors ... 181
A.2 Contact vs. Non-contact Descriptors ... 185

B Simulated Electrograms ... 189
B.1 Point-electrode Catheter ... 189
B.2 Modeled Catheter ... 192

References ... 195

List of Publications and Supervised Theses ... 211

List of Abbreviations

AF	Atrial Fibrillation
AFlut	Atrial Flutter
AP	Action Potential
APD	Action Potential Duration
AR	Activity Ratio
AS	Active Segment
AVC	Adaptive Ventricular Cancellation
CART	Classification and Regression Tree
CCP	Cost-Complexity-Pruning
CF	Characteristic Frequency
CFAE	Complex Fractionated Atrial Electrogram
CS	Coronary Sinus
DF	Dominant Frequency
DFT	Discrete Fourier Transformation
DWT	Discrete Wavelet Transformation
ECG	Electrocardiogram
EGM	Electrogram
EP	Electrophysiology
EPS	Entropy of Phase Space
EV	Eigenvalue
FDT	Fuzzy Decision Tree
FFT	Fast Fourier Transformation
GDI	Gini-Diversity-Index
ICA	Independent Component Analysis
IDFT	Inverse Discrete Fourier Transformation
IG	Information Gain
IGR	Information Gain Ratio
IQR	Interquartile Range
IVC	Inferior Vena Cava
IWT	Inverse Wavelet Transformation
LA	Left Atrium
LAA	Left Atrial Appendage

LIPV	Left Inferior Pulmonary Vein
LSPV	Left Superior Pulmonary Vein
LV	Left Ventricle
MAP	Monophasic Action Potential
MD	Medical Doctor
MLAS	Mean Length of Active Segments
MV	Mitral Valve
NLEO	Non-Linear Energy Operator
PC	Principle Component
PCA	Principle Component Analysis
PDF	Probability Density Function
PDS	Power Density Spectrum
PSSR	Phase Space Sample Ratio
PV	Pulmonary Vein
PVI	Pulmonary Vein Isolation
RA	Right Atrium
RIPV	Right Inferior Pulmonary Vein
RSPV	Right Superior Pulmonary Vein
RV	Right Ventricle
SD	Standard Deviation
SI	Split Information
STFT	Short Time Fourier Transformation
SVC	Superior Vena Cava
TMS	Template Matching and Subtraction
TV	Tricuspid Valve
VASR	Ventriculo-atrial Sample Ratio
VFF	Ventricular Far Field
WCT	Wilson Central Terminal
WT	Wavelet Transformation

1

Introduction

1.1 Motivation

Atrial fibrillation (AF) is the most common sustained supraventricular arrhythmia. The burden of AF rises with increasing age. Haemodynamic disorders and thromboembolic events caused by AF result in significant morbidity and mortality. In the western industrial nations approximately 1% of the adult population are suffering from AF. In Germany a population of nearly 1 million people are affected. In the last 20 years a rise of hospitalization of 66% could be determined. 1% of hospitalization is caused by AF. The social overall burden in Germany is approximately 3 billions € per year [1, 2]. So, there is keen interest in efficient and successful treatment of atrial fibrillation.

Catheter based radiofrequency ablation of AF has become a preferred method to treat AF. Although successful strategies exist to treat paroxysmal AF, the cure of persistant AF is still challenging. Physicians found different kinds of fractionated electrograms during ablation. Nademanee described "complex fractionated atrial electrograms" (CFAEs) as a parameter of the substrate of atrial fibrillation. Ablation of areas containing these CFAEs could terminate atrial fibrillation and may therefore play an important role in ablation strategies. AF ablation, therefore, is a signal guided process. Analyzing and interpreting atrial electrograms —especially high fractionated electrograms— is the basis of understanding the arrhythmia and planing the ablation procedure. The success rate of AF ablation is correlated strongly to the experience of the electrophysiologist.

Assisting physicians in analyzing CFAEs during ablation procedure is a challenging, but important topic to improve ablation success and reduce recurrence of AF. Improving medical experience gained from clinical practice can be done with signal processing and statistical methods. In this context several aspects are of special

importance. First, electrograms recorded during AF must be described in an objective and reproducible way. These descriptions must reflect the physiological behavior of the electrograms and the medical knowledge. Auxiliar new information might be provided by additional mathematical analysis. Second, the definition of complex fractionated atrial electrograms is ambiguous and each physician has an own understanding of these kind of signals. Hence, an automatic classification will assist the physicians and can guide unexperienced physicians. Third, newly gained information must be presented to the physicians in a way, that quick and easy interpreting is possible. 3D mapping systems currently used enable quick and easy visualization of patient specific atria with color coded information displayed on the surface. These systems can not be used for visualizing external data, as there is no uplink to these systems. Finally, the clinical outcome of new analyzing methods should be discussed with physicians and tested in a clinical environment. The discussion with physicians is an important step in inventing new methods, as the needs of clinical practice and the clinical utility have to be regarded.
To gain more insight into the mechanisms underlying persistent AF and to make the process of ablation of CFAEs more objective, signal processing and analysis of CFAEs are useful tools. Multivariate data analysis and statistics help to reproduce the physicians' view on signals in a mathematical way and provide methods to extend information and knowledge of the underlying mechanisms of AF. This way, additional computer based analysis of atrial electrograms could reduce examination times and improve success rates of AF ablation. Thus, the patients' burden and the overall treatment costs can be significantly reduced.

1.2 Aims of the Thesis

The major challenges in analyzing atrial electrograms, that are adressed in this thesis, are:

- Transposing the physician's view on atrial electrograms into mathematics and finding objective measures of clinical knowledge.
- Finding additional mathematical methods to investigate and measure features and attributes of complex fractionated atrial electrograms and visualize them on patient specific 3D anatomy.
- Automated classification of complex fractionated atrial electrograms into physiologically meaningful classes.

- Applying the new methods on clinical issues to push medical investigations of atrial fibrillation and complex fractionated atrial electrograms.

1.3 Structure of the Thesis

Part I introduces fundamental clinical and technical backgrounds:

Chapter 2 gives an overview of the medical background of the heart, atrial arrhythmias, and catheter ablation.

Chapter 3 introduces the used mathematical and signal processing methods.

Part II explains the methods and results, that were created and applied in this work:

Chapter 4 introduces atrial electrograms and describes signal preprocessing and the generated signal databases.

Chapter 5 shows a method to remove the ventricular far field from atrial electrograms.

Chapter 6 covers a method that divides atrial electrograms into active and inactive segments.

Chapter 7 introduces descriptors to explain and measure different features and attributes of atrial electrograms.

Chapter 8 displays a fuzzy decision tree to separate complex fractionated atrial electrograms into different classes.

Chapter 9 demonstrates an analysis of features of signals recorded with and without catheter contact to the atrial tissue. A comparison with simulated electrograms is performed and a decision tree is trained as classifier.

Chapter 10 displays how the newly gained information can be presented on a 3D model of patient specific atria.

Part III presents the application of created methods on clinical issues:

Chapter 11 analyzes the influence of different atrial rhythms on the complexity of atrial electrograms.

Chapter 12 discusses the influence of pulmonary vein isolation on the fractionation distribution of atrial electrograms.

Chapter 13 presents a discussion on finding continuous activity within highly fractionated electrogram distribution.

Part IV presents additional results:

Appendix A displays descriptor results calculated on the CFAE database and descriptor results calculated on the contact/non-contact database.

Appendix B covers additional results from simulated electrograms.

Finally, chapter 14 summarizes the thesis and gives an outlook on possible future work.

Part I

Basic Foundations

2

Medical Background

2.1 Anatomy and Physiology of the Heart

The human heart is a muscular hollow organ, which is placed in the anterior, inferior part of the mediastinum between the lungs and above the diaphragm. Due to its placement the heart changes its position and orientation according to the breathing movements of the lungs, diaphragm, and ribs. The heart weight of an adult man averages 320 g, of an adult woman 280 g depending on the age. The filling volume of the heart is between 250 ml and 400 ml [3,4].

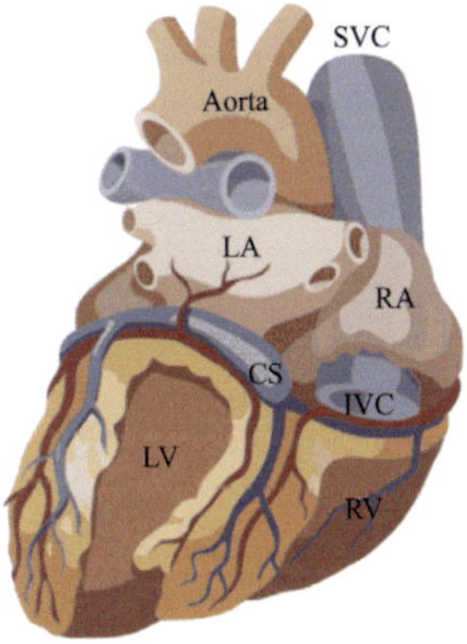

Fig. 2.1: The heart, adapted from [5]. LA, left atrium; RA, right atrium; LV, left ventricle; RV, right ventricle; SVC, superior vena cava; IVC, inferior vena cava; CS, coronary sinus.

The heart acts as a pump for the circulatory system. It is responsible for pumping blood through the vessels by repeated, rhythmic contraction and relaxation. The human heart is composed of four chambers, two superior atria and two inferior ventricles. The atria are responsible for receiving blood and filling the ventricles. The ventricles are the discharging chambers. Functionally, the heart consists of two parts which are separated by the cardiac septum. The left heart (left atrium (LA) and ventricle (LV)) pumps blood through the systemic circuit and the right heart (right atrium (RA) and ventricle (RV)) pumps the blood through the pulmonary circuit.

Venous blood from the systemic circuit is collected by the inferior vena cava (IVC) and superior vena cava (SVC) and directed into the right atrium. The blood gets through the tricuspid valve to the right ventricle. From here the blood is pumped through the pulmonary valve via the pulmonary artery into the lungs. In the pulmonary circulation the deoxygenated blood is enriched with oxygen. It returns from the lungs through the pulmonary veins to the left atrium where it is pumped through the mitral (bicuspid) valve into the left ventricle before leaving through the aortic valve to the aorta [3].

The wall of the heart consists of three layers. The endocardium is the inner layer, which covers the whole interior. The outer layer is called epicardium and is simultaneously the inner layer of the pericardium (inner serous pericardium). The myocardium is located between the endocardium and the epicardium and is responsible for the contraction and performance of the heart [3]. The myocardium in the four chambers is built up of smooth muscles and variable thickness. Atrial myocardium is significantly thinner than ventricular myocardium. Also the myocardium of the right ventricle is significantly thinner than the left myocardium as the pressure in the right ventricle is $25-30\,\text{mmHg}$ and in the left ventricle $120-150\,\text{mmHg}$.

The heart is surrounded by a pericardial sac (pericardium). The pericardium is divided into two layers: the outermost fibrous pericardium and the inner serous pericardium. The serous pericardium, in turn, is divided into the parietal pericardium and the visceral pericardium, which is part of the epicardium. A thin film of fluid lubricates the space between the parietal and visceral pericardial layers (pericardial cavity). Thus, a frictionless motion of the heart is possible.

2.2 Electrophysiological Basics

The heart has two different types of cells: Conduction cells that build and forward impulses and cells that respond to an impulse with a contraction (myocytes). The myocytes build a functional syncytium: all cells are non-insulated. That means that an impulse anywhere in the myocardium will lead to a complete contraction of the heart. The excitation of the heart physiologically starts at the sinoatrial node (SA node, sinus node), which acts as a physiological, autonomous pacemaker. The excitation spreads over the atria and the atrioventricular node (AV node), to the bundles of His and the Purkinje fibres, which transfer the excitation to the myocardium. In the AV node the excitation is delayed to optimize the filling of the ventricles (fig. 2.2) [3,4].

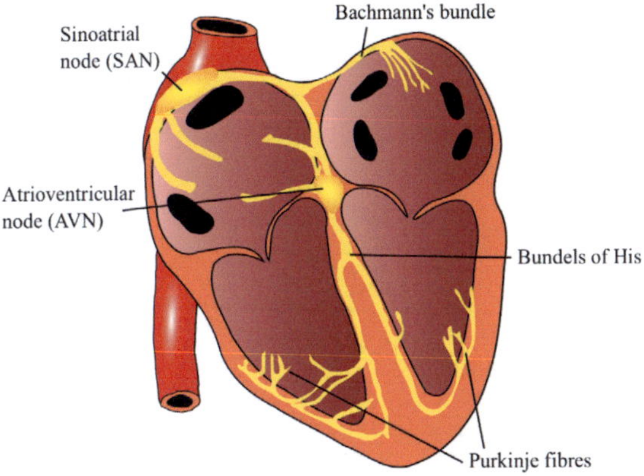

Fig. 2.2: Conduction system of the human heart, adapted from [6].

If an excitable cell (nervous or muscle cell) is irritated by an impulse, the ion conductivity of its membran is changing. If the stimulus is strong enough to excite the cell, the cell reacts with an action potential (AP, fig. 2.3). This AP represents the forwarded signal in a nerve and leads to a contraction in a muscular cell. In an unexcited state the resting potential between the intracellular space and the extracellular space across the cell's membrane (transmembrane voltage) is −90 mV. This potential is caused by different concentrations of ions in the intra- and extracellular space. The resting potential is increased towards 0 mV by the stimulus. If the transmembrane voltage reaches a threshold around −60 mV, sodium channels in the membran are opened and sodium is flowing into the intracellular space. This influx of electrical positive ions causes the AP to collapse rapidly (depolarization). The change of the transmembrane voltage causes the potassium and calcium channels to open, what leads to a decrease of the transmembrane voltage. Unique to myocardial cells is an inflow of calcium into the intracellular space. This leads to a delayed repolarization, called the plateau phase. In this plateau phase, the cell is unexcitable again until the transmembrane voltage reaches approximately $-20\,\mathrm{mV}$. This phase is called absolute refractory period. In the following relative refractory period the transmembrane voltage is decreased by an inward potassium current and the cell is excitable again, but will react to a stimulus with an AP of lower height and rate of rise. When the resting potential is reached again, the former ion concentration and distribution is recovered (fig. 2.3) [3,6].

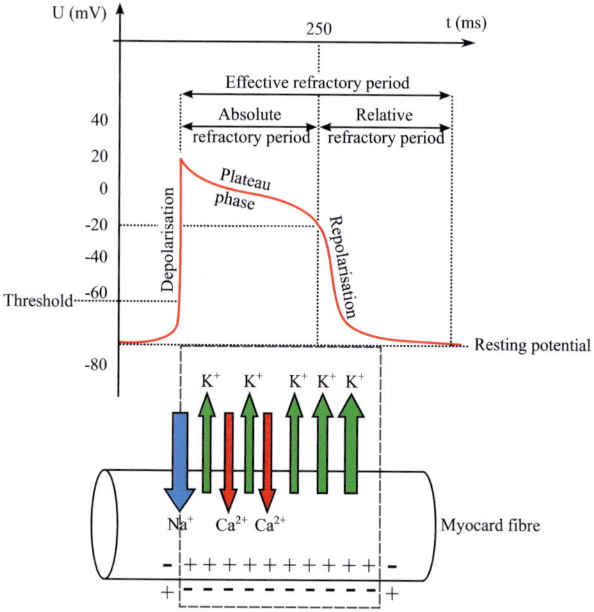

Fig. 2.3: Action potential of the myocardium, adapted from [7].

Each AP in the sinus node initiates a heart beat, and thus the SA node is the generator of normal sinus rhythm (fig. 2.7). If the SA node does not generate an initial impulse, or the impulse generated in the SA node is blocked, usually the atrioventricular node will take control of the heart's rhythm. If the AV node also fails, the bundle of His or the Purkinje fibers are also capable of acting as the pacemaker.

The atrioventricular node as well as the bundle of His or the Purkinje fibres do not normally control the heart rate because their pacemaker frequency is lower than the SA node frequency. Thus, the excitation originating from the SA node reaches the subjacent pacemaker centres before their spontaneous depolarization reaches their own threshold potential.
The atrioventricular node also has the property of decremental conduction [8]. The more frequently the node is stimulated the slower it conducts. So, it is acting as a frequency filter. The AV node prevents rapid conduction to the ventricle in cases of rapid atrial rhythms, such as atrial fibrillation or atrial flutter, that could otherwise lead to ventricular fibrillation and cardiac arrest [4, 6].
With help of the electrocardiogram (ECG) the potential differences originating from the electrical activity from the heart can be visualized. The ECG provides information about the rate and regularity of heartbeats as well as the size and position of the chambers, the presence of any damage to the heart, and the effect of drugs. The potentials emerge on the border zone between excited and non-excited myocardium. As the excitation propagates across the myocardium, manifold potentials that differ in size arise. The summation of these manifold small potentials can be measured as summarized potential on the body's surface. Electrodes are placed on the body surface and the amplified potential difference is recorded by an ECG recorder. The ECG is a projection of the spatial cardiac activity on the axis between the electrodes (fig. 2.4).
A physiological normal ECG curve (fig. 2.5) consists of the following parts:

- P wave: depolarization of atria in response to a SA node trigger
- PR interval: delay of AV node to allow filling of ventricles
- QRS complex: depolarization of ventricles, triggers main pumping contractions
- ST segment: beginning of ventricle repolarization
- T wave: ventricular repolarization

Conventional leads to measure the ECG are the leads defined by Einthoven [10], Goldberger [11, 12], and Wilson [13, 14]. The Einthoven leads are bipolar leads. The voltage between the right arm (R), the left arm (L), and the left leg (L) are measured (I, II, III, fig. 2.4). Goldberger used the same electrode locations to achieve an ECG. But in contrast to Einthoven, Goldberger measured the voltage between one lead and the remaining two leads interconnected via a resistor (aVR, aVL, aVF, fig. 2.4). In addition to these 6 leads Wilson defined another 6 electrode positions on the chest in close proximity to the heart. The voltage is measured between

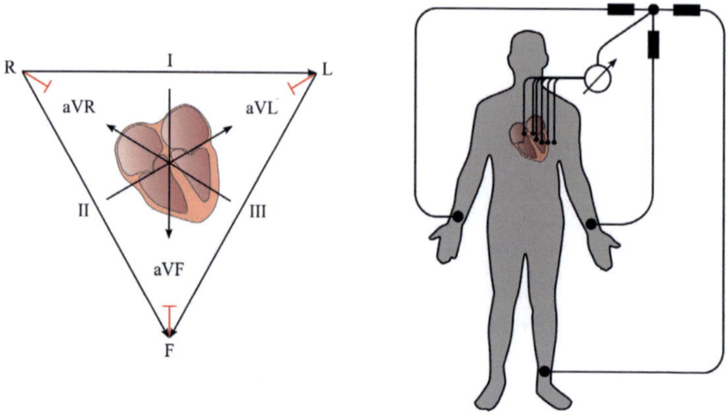

Fig. 2.4: Standard ECG leads. Einthoven (I, II, III) and Goldberger (aVR, aVL, aVF) leads are depicted on the left hand side. Wilson leads are depicted on the right hand side, adapted from [9].

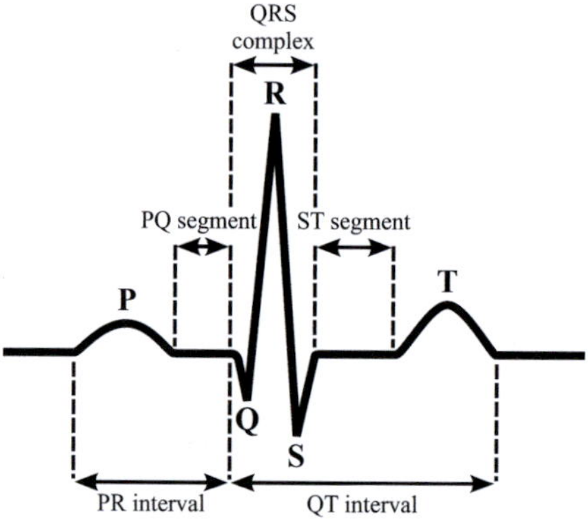

Fig. 2.5: Schematic representation of a normal ECG.

one of the chest electrodes and the Wilson's central terminal (WCT) as reference electrode. Wilson's central terminal is produced by connecting the electrodes, R, L, and F via a simple resistive network to give an average potential across the body, which approximates the potential at infinity. Nowadays this resistive network is replaced by high impedance amplifieres to avoid a current draw by the voltage measurement circuit.

2.3 The Atria & Atrial Arrhythmias

The purpose of the right and the left atrium is to act as a collecting tank and to fill the right respectively the left ventricle with blood. The right atrium receives deoxygenated blood from the superior vena cava (SVC), inferior vena cava (IVC) and coronary sinus (CS). The left atrium receives oxygenated blood from the left superior (LSPV), the left inferior (LIPV), the right superior (RSPV) and the right inferior (RIPV) pulmonary veins (fig. 2.6). The tricuspid valve (TV) between the right atrium and the right ventricle prevents blood flowing back into the atrium when the ventricle contracts. The mitral valve (MV) between the left atrium and left ventricle has the same purpose for the left atrium and the left ventricle.

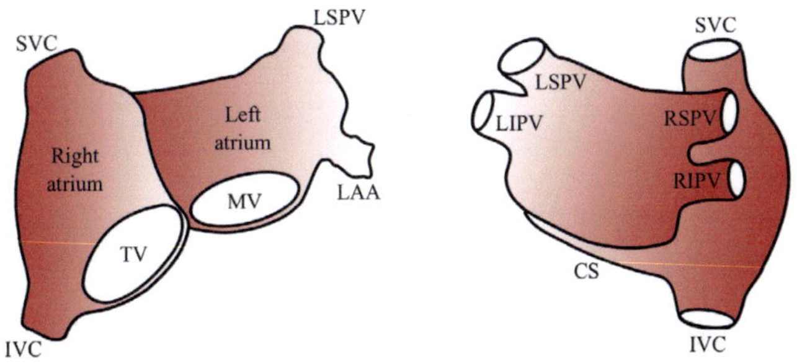

(a) Anterior-posterior view (b) Posterior-anterior view

Fig. 2.6: Left and right atria, adapted from [15]. SVC, superior vena cava; IVC, inferior vena cava; TV, tricuspid valve; MV, mitral valve; LAA, left atrial appendage; LSPV, left superior pulmonary vein; LIPV, left inferior pulmonary vein; RSPV, right superior pulmonary vein; RIPV, right inferior pulmonary vein; CS, coronary sinus.

The fossa ovalis, found in the right atrium, is an embryonic remnant of the foramen ovale, which normally closes shortly after birth. It is a shallow pit between the right and left atrium. The foramen ovale is a door-like connection between the atria that enables the transfer of blood from the right to the left fetal heart circuit. The fossa ovalis has importance for the ablation of AF in the left atrium as it is used as port for a catheter from the right to the left atrium.

Modifications or alteration of physiological pathways for excitation can lead to severe complications and malfunctions of the heart or parts of the heart. Often the heart rate is influenced by these processes. Deseases that influence or change the heart rate are called arrhythmias. A cardiac arrhythmia is an electrical cardiac activity, that is characterized by an irregular sequence of excitations, a change of the regular heart frequency of 60 – 100 beats per minute, or a disorder of the temporal process of cardiac activity. An arrhythmia that is slower than 60 beats per minute is called bradycardia, if it is faster than 100 beats per minute in physical rest it is called tachycardia.

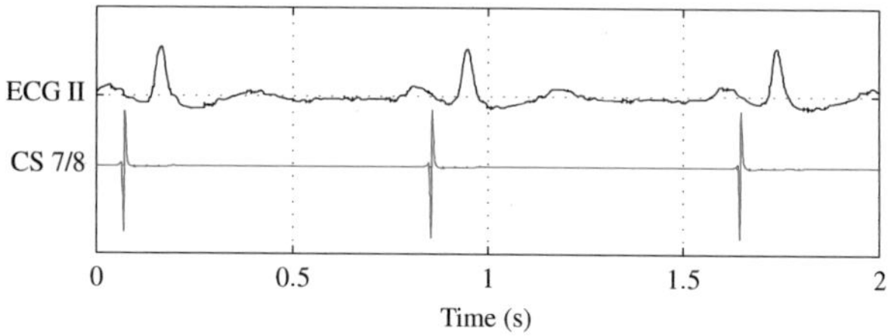

Fig. 2.7: Surface ECG and atrial electrogram during sinus rhythm. The EGM was measured in the coronary sinus.

The regular physiological heart rhythm is called sinus rhythm (fig. 2.7). An atrial tachycardia is a fast rhythm disorder of the atria. The most prominent atrial tachycardias are atrial flutter and atrial fibrillation.

2.3.1 Atrial Flutter

Atrial Flutter (AFlut) is a tachycardiac arrhythmia of the atria originating from a reentry mechanism. AFlut appears often paroxysmally, seldom chronically and can change into atrial fibrillation. In the electrocardiogram (ECG) AFlut is recognized with a strongly increased but regular atrial frequency (200 – 350 beats per minute) and fast sequential, broadened, and often sawtooth-shaped P waves (fig. 2.8). AFlut is caused by various cardiac diseases (e.g. ischemia, myocarditis, cardiomyopathy, valvular diseases, etc.), but can also occur after heart surgery or after ablation of AF. Very rarely it can occur idiopathic in healthy people. Symptoms are mainly caused by the high heart frequency (dyspnea, bodily weakness, syncope, . . .). The risk of developing a thrombus is given, especially during permanent AFlut, and is similar compared with AF. AFlut can be treated medically with antiarrhythmic drugs, with electric cardioversion, or preferentially with catheter ablation [16].

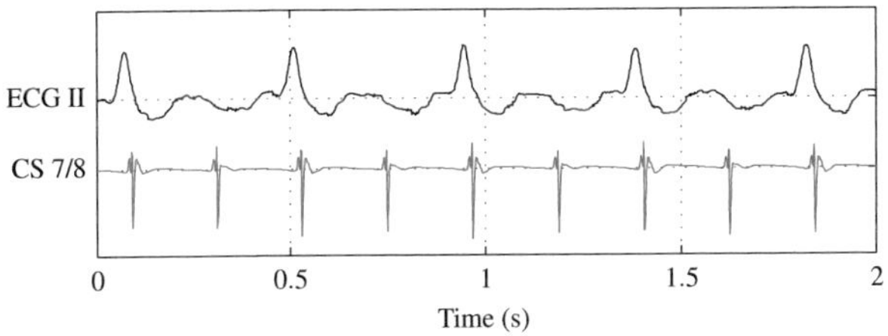

Fig. 2.8: Surface ECG and atrial electrogram during atrial flutter. The EGM was measured in the coronary sinus.

2.3.2 Atrial Fibrillation

Definition

Atrial Fibrillation (AF) is a supraventricular tachyarrhythmia. AF is characterized by an uncoordinated atrial activity, that leads to a continuous impairment of the mechanical atrial function. During atrial fibrillation the atria are depolarized with a frequency of 350 – 600 beats per minute. In the electrocardiogram the P wave during AF is substituted by a fast oscillation or a fibrillating wave with varying amplitude and shape. The ventricular contraction is irregular and frequently increased presuming unimpaired atrio-ventricular excitation.

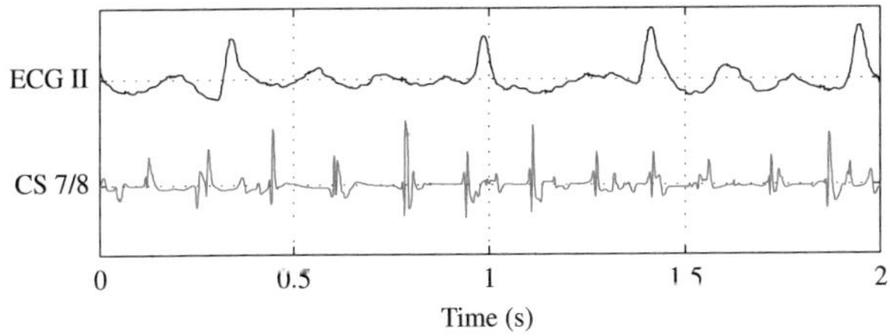

Fig. 2.9: Surface ECG and atrial electrogram during atrial fibrillation. The EGM was measured in the coronary sinus.

Classification

The different types of atrial fibrillation have been divided in an international unified nomenclature [1, 17, 18]. A differentiation is made between:

- **Paroxysmal atrial fibrillation**: more than 2 episodes of AF, that last less than 7 days and terminate spontaneously.
- **Persistent atrial fibrillation**: AF, that sustains longer then 7 days, does not terminate spontaneously, but can be terminated with direct-current cardioversion or with pharmacological therapy. After a cardioversion sinus rhythm persists for several days to months. Does the fibrillation period sustain longer than a year, it is called *"long-standing persistent atrial fibrillation"*.
- **Permanent atrial fibrillation**: AF, that terminates neither with electrical nor with pharmacological cardioversion.

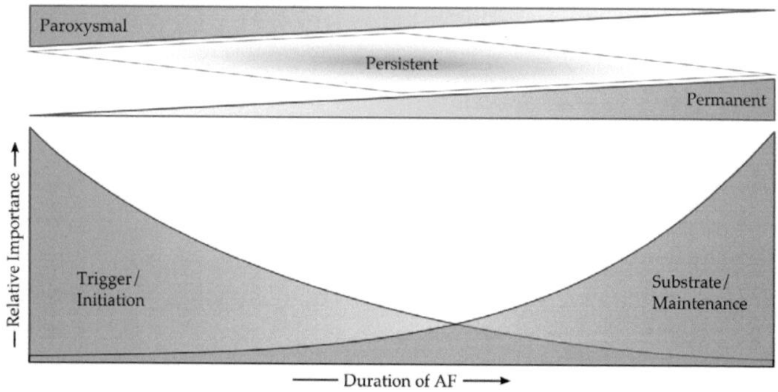

Fig. 2.10: The influence of trigger and substrate on atrial fibrillation. AF is divided into three categories. Paroxysmal AF is mainly a trigger based process, whereas permanent AF is substrate dependent. Persistent AF is a mixture of trigger based and remodeling of the substrate based processes, adapted from [19, 20].

Epidemiology and Prognosis

Atrial Fibrillation is the most common perpetuating tachycardia in the adult population. In the western industrial nations $1-2\%$ of the total population is suffering from AF. The number of people suffering from AF will be doubled within the next two to three decades, if not to be increased threefold [1, 21, 22]. Studies showed, that the risk factors for the development of AF are increasing age, hypertension, heart failure, valve disease, and coronary artery disease. Thus, $5-10\%$ of the 60-year-old and 20% of the 85-year-old are diseased with AF [23–25]. In the Framingham Heart Study it could be proven, that atrial fibrillation doubles mortality independent of comorbidity [26, 27]. With existing comorbidity, mortality rises. Mortality rises a 2.4-fold with coincident coronary heart disease [28]. The risk of a stroke with underlying AF is between 1.5% and 24%, depending on the age [22,29].

Socio-economic Meaning

Due to risen life expectation, the growing prevalence of chronic cardiac diseases and increased usage of screening- and ambulant monitoring-systems, diagnostics and treatment of AF is a substantial burden of the financial and personal resources of the public health care system [30]. Within the last 20 years there was a rise of 66% of hospitalization [31–33]. In the USA as well as in Germany approximately 1% of hospitalization is caused by atrial fibrillation [2, 30]. The costs of clinical care of AF sum up of hospital costs (52%), costs of medication (23%), follow-up (9%), follow-up examinations (8%), disability (6%) and emergency measures (2%) [34]. The annual costs per patient amount to 3000 € approximately. This indicates, that the social overall burden is huge (entire EU: 13.5 billions € for 4.5 millions ill people [1]) and will rather be escalating in the coming years than decrease.

Pathophysiologic Mechanisms

The pathophysiology of AF is complex and not completely understood yet. Genetic predisposition, structural change and fibrosis, progression of cardiac diseases, inflammation, autonomous dysfunction paired with electrophysiological abnormality of the atria and pulmonary veins (PV), promote occurrence and maintenance of AF. Early experimental studies and computer models seemed to suggest multiple reentry-waves as origin of AF. With proceeding advances in mapping technologies and their usage during open heart surgery or during electrophysiological studies, stable as well as non-stable reentry-circles with short cycle length within or in close proximity to the pulmonary veins could be identified as cause for AF [1, 17]. To the current state of research AF is caused by the following mechanisms [1,17]:

Multiple Wavelet Hypothesis Until the end of the 1980s the multiple wavelet hypothesis was considered the cause of AF. According to this hypothesis AF origins by the presence of parallel existing micro-reentry-circles (fig. 2.11(a)) in the left and right atria [35]. In this model self-exciting fibrillating areas are depending on the conduction velocity of the tissue, the refractory period and tissue mass. AF is benefitted by slow conduction velocity, a shortened refractory period and increased tissue mass. From this model the maze-surgery was developed as therapy of AF [36, 37].

Focal Trigger Focal trigger (fig. 2.11(b)) as cause of AF could be observed during electrophysiological studies very early. Haissaguerre could show for the first time, that focal trigger originating from the pulmonary veins can introduce AF [38]. He could also show, that ablation of the source trigger could terminate the AF [38–42]. This serves as a proof, that AF can be induced by a focal trigger and that by eliminating or isolating this trigger the AF can be terminated. This applies particularly for paroxysmal AF and leads to different kinds of ablation lines for the catheter ablation procedure [42–47].

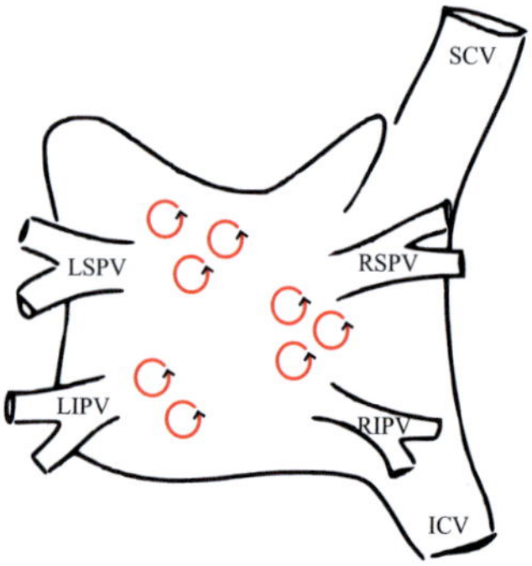

(a) Multi-wavelets as trigger and maintenance of AF.

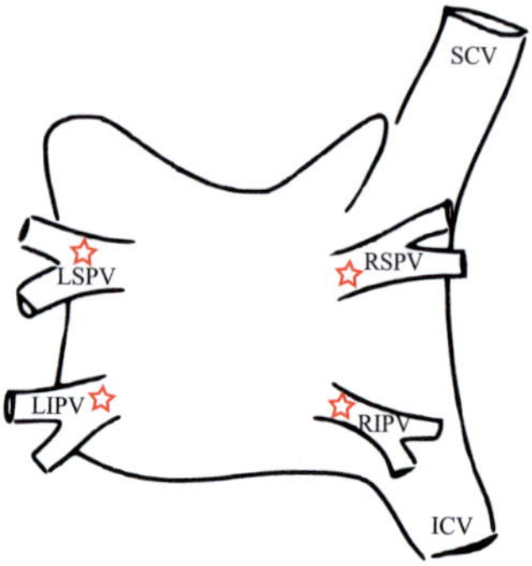

(b) Focal triggers originating from the pulmonary veins.

Fig. 2.11: Possible causes of atrial fibrillation, adapted from [48].

Electric Remodeling In the case of persistent AF sinus rhythm can be restored in a high percentage with an electric cardioversion. Regarding the long-term success rate it becomes clear, that a cardioversion of AF, less than 24 hour duration, had a notable higher success rate and lower recurrence rate than AF with more than 24 hour. Following these examinations the thesis "Atrial fibrillation begets atrial fibrillation" was verbalized [49]. Consequently several scientists searched for cellular and electrical mechanism to explain this phenomenon. They found that the AF itself can influence the expression of ionic channels of the myocytes and can therefore modify the electrical characteristics of these cells. The extremely fast excitation of the atria during atrial fibrillation are leading to a shortened AP, a shortened refractory period with a high frequency adaption and a reduced cycle length, which again rises the risk of reentry circles [49, 50] (fig. 2.12). Likewisc increased atrial

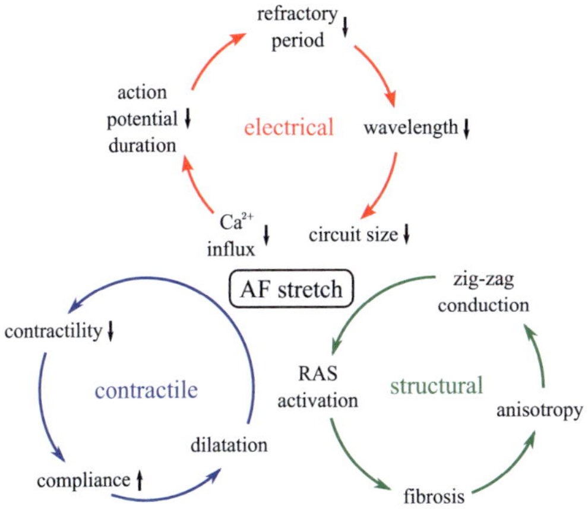

Fig. 2.12: Positive feedback-loops of remodeling during atrial fibrillation, adapted from [51].

pressure in case of structural cardiac diseases, arterial hypertension, aging and genetic variations lead to continuous structural atrial modifications [52–55]. These processes lead to an increased incidence of AF. The electro-anatomic substrate is characterized by a non-uniform anisotropy, local heterogeneity of conduction and slowed excitation propagation [51, 56–58].

Autonomous Nerve System of the Atria Bettoni et al. could show, that an increase of the sympathetic and the parasympathetic tonus precede the beginning of paroxysmal AF [59]. These findings were also verified by other studies [60, 61]. Spontaneous "firing" of the pulmonary veins followed by AF can be introduced by an electric stimulation of the ganglionic plexi or the autonomous nerve endings, which activate retrogradely the ganglia [62]. A result from this experimental study is the hypothesis, that the intrinsic cardiac autonomous nervous system promotes the development of triggered AF.

2.4 Catheter Ablation of Atrial Fibrillation

Beside the medical treatment, catheter ablation has become more and more an alternative treatment for symptomatic AF. For ablation the RF energy and the cryo-energy are available [63]. Up to now, the technique of the isolation of the pulmonary veins is the only curative treatment for patients with paroxsysmal AF [64, 65]. The endpoint of most AF studies is therefore freedom of atrial fibrillation without antiarrhythmic drugs [66]. Catheter ablation is performed during electrophysiological (EP) studies and is a signal driven method. Therefore, different types of electrode catheters are inserted via venous access and are placed at distinctive locations in the heart such as the sinus node, the PVs or inside the coronary sinus to analyze atrial electrograms and to get an idea of the cardiac excitation and its malfunction.

2.4.1 Catheter Ablation

The aim of a catheter ablation is to isolate ectopic triggers within the pulmonary veins or in the atrial substrate. Whereas the technique of the pulmonary vein isolation is well established, the modification of the atrial substrate by RF energy is less established and mainly driven by the physicians experience. Therefore, an ablation catheter is introduced via the femoral vein into the right atrium (fig. 2.14(a)). To access the left atrium and the pulmonary veins a transseptal puncture has to be performed. The safest location to cross from the right to the left atrium is the fossa ovalis. Once the catheters are positioned at the right spot, ablation can be started (fig. 2.14(b)).

Radio-frequency ablation uses the heat generated from a high frequency alternating current to ablate tissue. During RF ablation, high-frequency currents with 300 to 1000 kHz are inserted into the tissue at the tip of an ablation catheter (fig. 2.13(a)). An advantage of high frequency current is that it does not directly stimulate nerves or the heart muscle. Usually, a unipolar setup is used with a large ground electrode at the patient's back. The high density of electric current near the catheter tip causes local resistive heating of the tissue in a 2 mm radius [65]. Deeper regions in the myocardial wall are progressively heated due to thermal conduction [67]. The tissue must be heated up to at least 50° C, to destroy myocardial cells and set non-conducting lesions in the tissue. However, temperatures should not trespass 70° C to reduce the dangers of thromboembolic complications.

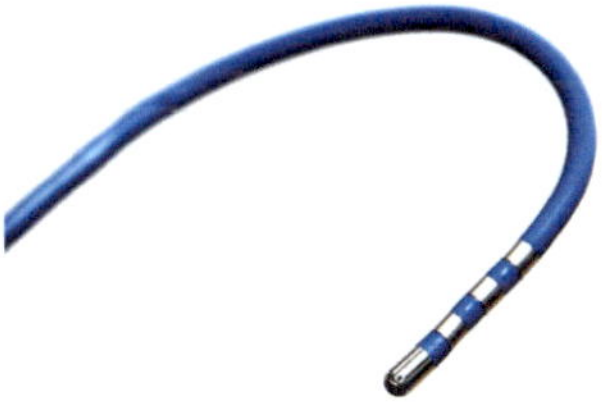

(a) A typical 4-pole ablation catheter with equidistant spaced electrodes. The tip electrode at the distal end of the catheter is 4 mm, all other electrodes are 2 mm. The inter-electrode spacing is 2 mm.

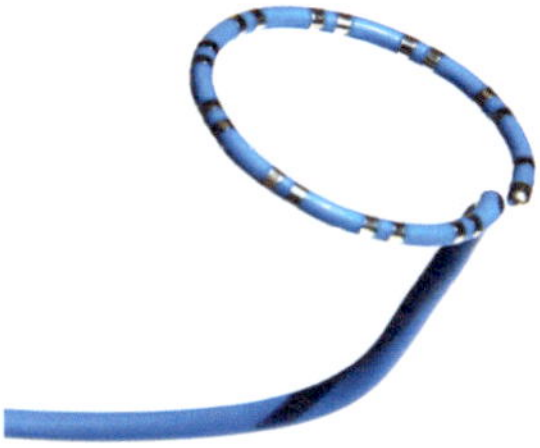

(b) A multi-polar circular mapping catheter. The electrodes have a width of 1 mm and the inter-electrode spacing is 1 mm and 4 mm, respectively.

Fig. 2.13: Two examples of common catheters used during catheter ablation. The straight catheter on the left is used for ablation as well as for analyzing EGMs. The circular catheter on the right is a typical analyzing catheter that gives spatial information about the tachycardia.

Therefore, tip temperature and impedance are constantly monitored during the ablation process. To avoid local temperature peaks at the electrode tip, irrigated tip electrodes are used [65]. To ensure not only superficial but also transmural lesions, ablation currents are typically applied for 60 s to set an ablation point.

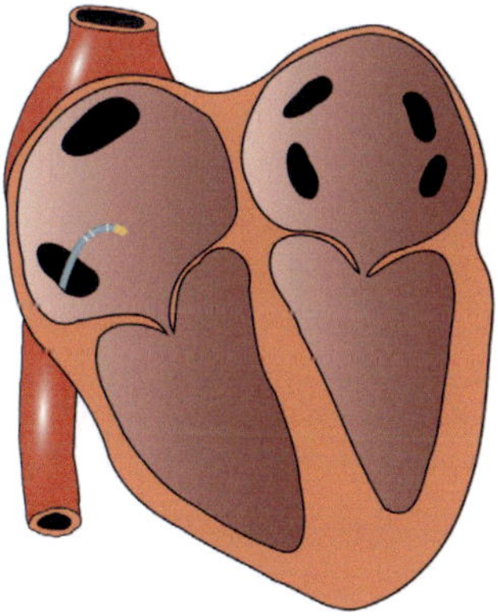

(a) The ablation catheter is pushed via the inferior vena cava into the right atrium.

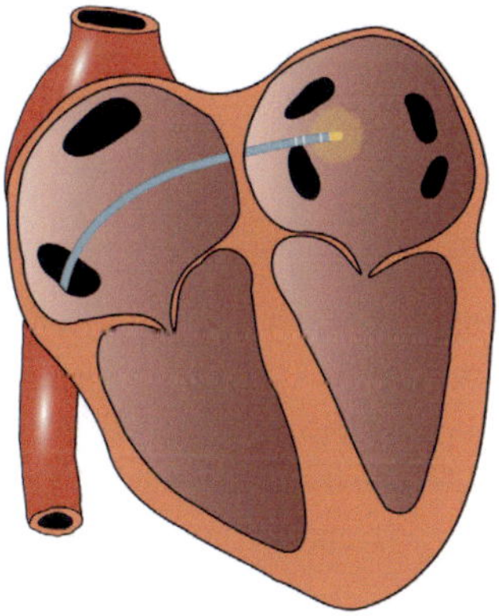

(b) Crossing the intra-atrial septum, irregular tissue can be destroyed by use of electrical energy.

Fig. 2.14: Radio-frequency catheter ablation. Displayed is a typical ablation catheter with four electrodes.

Cryoablation instead is less flexible but easier to handle. Typically, cryoablation is used as an alternative way to isolate the pulmonary veins. In opposite to the radio-frequency ablation cryoablation cools down the tissue to –80° C to destroy irregular cells or electrically isolate triggers within the pulmonary veins.

2.4.2 Mapping

To know exactly at which position the catheter is at any time of the examination, fluoroscopy is used regularly. Fluoroscopy provides only two-dimensional representation of the atrium and does not relate local electrograms to their spatial orientation. In addition X-rays are noxious for the patient as well as the physicians and nurses. To overcome these shortcomings 3D electroanatomical mapping systems are used to reduce the amount of X-rays and provide the physician with 3D location of catheters and measured electrograms. The most common anatomical mapping systems used in the clinical setup at the moment are the EnSite NavX™ (St. Jude Medical, St. Paul, MN, USA) and CARTO (Biosense Webster, Diamond Bar, CA, USA). Both systems use deflectable catheters which are available in various sizes and various realizations (fig. 2.13). Most common catheters are circular mapping catheters (10-pole or 14-pole), a straight 4-pole ablation catheter and an 8-pole straight catheter as reference in the coronary sinus. Other catheters are the 5-armed catheter (PENTARAY, Biosense Webster) or the spiral shaped catheters (e.g. AFocus II, St. Jude Medical).

The CARTO system features an ultra low magnetic field emitter and a miniature passive magnetic field sensor embedded in the distal electrode of the catheter (fig. 2.15(a)). The magnetic field emitters are placed under the operating table beneath the patient's thorax [65]. The magnetic field decreases in strength and changes direction as a function of distance. The position of each coil is measured beforehand and thus the position of the catheter can be estimated by quantifying the intensity and direction of all three magnetic fields. Also the orientation of the catheter can be determined.

The EnSite NavX™ system is an impedance based system: It uses the electrodes of the catheters to sense a 5.68 kHz low current signal which is coupled into the body by three pairs of large electrodes. These electrodes are placed on the patient's thorax to create transthoracic orthogonal electric fields with the heart at its center (fig. 2.15(b)) [68]. The fields are measured with a sampling rate of 93 Hz and thus allow a location in almost real time [65].

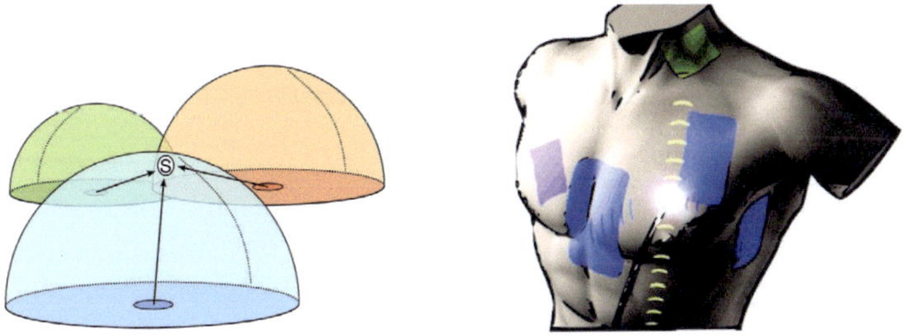

(a) CARTO: Magnetic field based localisation of the catheter tip.

(b) EnSite NavX™: Impedance based localisation of catheter electrodes.

Fig. 2.15: Basic principles of CARTO and EnSite NavX™ mapping systems, adapted from [65, 69]

These systems provide a method to localize at least the tip-electrode of the ablation catheter (CARTO) or all electrodes of any catheter plugged into the system (EnSite NavX™). If the catheter is moved over the endocard of the atrium, the catheter locations are tracked and from this point cloud the surface of the atrium can be computed (fig. 2.16). In a second step this surface can be registered with a 3D anatomy gained from a CT scan or a MRI scan.

Also the measurement position for each electrogram recorded by the catheter is known. Thus, a colored map with information provided by analysis of the electrograms can be visualized.

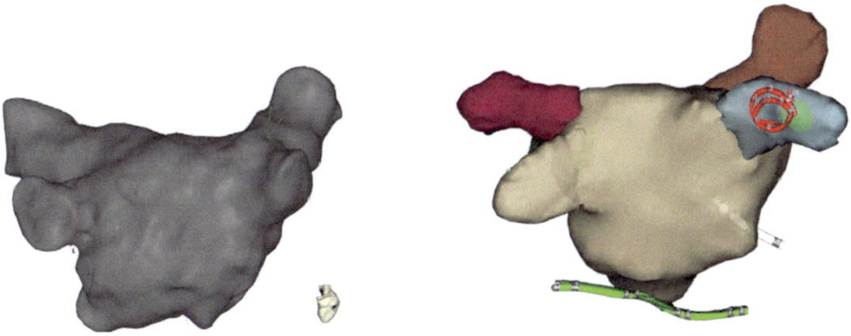

(a) CARTO map

(b) EnSite NavX™ map

Fig. 2.16: Anatomical maps resulting from moving a catheter over the endocard of the left atrium (posterior view).

2.5 Cell Modeling

The development of models of cellular dynamics and of realistic anatomical structures enables computer simulations to become an important tool for the investigation of cardiac excitation propagation and arrhythmia. Computer models of the heart can also be used to analyze the influence of electrodes, catheters or interventional methods (e.g. catheter ablation lesions) on the endocardium. Basis of all these simulations is the transformation of dynamic processes of a singular cell into a system of coupled differential equations. The cell model includes transmembrane voltage, ionic currents, and the ion concentrations. A tissue model is based on the cell model and describes the geometric structure of the tissue to allow for the electrical interconnections between cells.

2.5.1 Hodgkin-Huxley Model

Hodgkin and Huxley were the first to model membrane kinetics of an excitable cell (neuron) in 1952 [70]. They delivered a mathematical description for the ionic mechanisms underlying electrophysiological phenomena. Their model is based on the results of voltage-clamp experiments on axons of the giant squid. In this model, the electric current across the cell membrane during activation is described by a net of parallel changeable conductors (fig. 2.17).

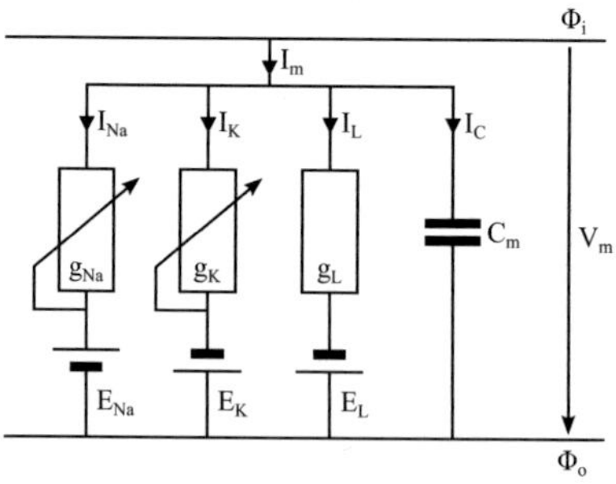

Fig. 2.17: An electric circuit representation of the Hodgkin-Huxley model (adapted from [6]).

The membrane's lipid bilayer is represented as a capacitance C_m. Voltage-gated ion channels are represented by nonlinear electrical conductances g_k (k is the specific ion). The linear conductance g_L represents leak channels. The electrochemical gradients driving the flow of ions are represented by batteries E_k and E_L, the values of which are determined from the Nernst potential of the specific ion. The currents I_{Na}, I_K, and I_L arise from the difference of the membrane voltage V_m and the particular resting voltage E_k (Nernst voltage) and the appropriate conductance g_k (eq. (2.1)).

$$I_k = (V_m - E_k) \cdot g_k \qquad E_k = \frac{\mathrm{R}T}{z_k\mathrm{F}} \ln \frac{c_{k,i}}{c_{k,o}} \tag{2.1}$$

The Nernst equation can be used to calculate the voltage E_k of an ion k of charge z across a membrane. This potential difference is determined using the concentration of the ion inside ($c_{k,i}$) and outside ($c_{k,o}$) the cell (R ideal gas constant, F Faraday's constant, T temperature). The total transmembrane current density is described as the sum of the capacitive and ionic components [70]

$$\begin{aligned} I_m &= I_C + I_{Na} + I_K + I_L \\ &= C_m \frac{dV_m}{dt} + (V_m - E_{Na})g_{Na} + (V_m - E_K)g_K + (V_m - E_L)g_L, \end{aligned} \tag{2.2}$$

where

I_m = membrane current
C_m = membrane capacitance
V_m = membrane voltage
E_{Na}, E_K, E_L = Nernst voltage for Na^+, K^+ and leakage ions
g_{Na}, g_K, g_L = membrane conductance for Na^+, K^+ and leakage ions.

Ion channels in the cell membrane can be opened or closed. This behavior is time and voltage dependent and can be modeled with gating variables. These gating variables calculate the probability p whether a gate is open p or not $1-p$. The Na^+-channel consists of three independent but identical activating m gates and one inactivating h gate, whereas the K^+-channel is build from four activating n gates. Thus, the conductivity results in

$$g_{Na} = g_{Na,\max} m^3 h \tag{2.3}$$

$$g_K = g_{K,\max} n^4. \tag{2.4}$$

The transition between the open and closed state for the gating variables are controlled by voltage dependent rate constants α and β that change with time while V_m is changing. The probability to get to an open state is described by α, the probability to get to a closed state is described by β. Their time-depending behavior can be described by

$$\begin{aligned}\dot{m} &= \alpha_m(1-m) - \beta_m m \\ \dot{h} &= \alpha_h(1-h) - \beta_h h \\ \dot{n} &= \alpha_n(1-n) - \beta_n n.\end{aligned} \tag{2.5}$$

The Hodgkin-Huxley model can be extended to more cell properties, e.g. further ion channels, or it can be adapted to other cell idiosyncrasies or pathologies. The Hodgkin-Huxley model is, therefore, commonly used as a basis for more complex cell models.

2.5.2 Courtemanche-Ramirez-Nattel Model

The Courtemanche-Ramirez-Nattel (CRN) model is a mathematical model of an atrial human cell, based on the Hodgkin-Huxley cell model [71]. It describes the electrical behavior of a cell with a set of nonlinear-coupled ordinary differential equations. This model takes ion concentrations, ionic currents, and bindings to intracellular structures into account. It is used in this work to simulate atrial electrograms (chapter 9). The transmembrane voltage of the CRN model is given by

$$V_m = \frac{dV}{dt} = \frac{-(I_m + I_{st})}{C_m}, \tag{2.6}$$

where I_m is the total membrane current and I_{st} is an external stimulus current. I_m is the sum of 12 ionic currents:

$$I_m = I_{Na} + I_{K1} + I_{to} + I_{Kur} + I_{Kr} + I_{Ks} + I_{Ca,L} + I_{p,Ca} + I_{NaK} + I_{NaCa} + I_{b,Na} + I_{b,Ca}. \tag{2.7}$$

Table 2.1 gives a more detailed overview of the different currents and their definition. A schematic representation of the Courtemanche-Ramirez-Nattel cell model with all currents, pumps and exchangers is depicted in figure 2.18. The model constants are given in table 2.2.

The CRN model allows for time varying intracellular ion distribution of Na^+, K^+, and Ca^{2+} in addition to the ion channels and their specific gating variables, which are an extension of the Hodgkin-Huxley model. Furthermore, the bearings of junctional sarcoplasmic reticulum (JSR) and the network sarcoplasmic reticulum (NSR) are incorporated. Cytoplasm, SJR and NSR are realized as individual

Table 2.1: Components of I_m based on the model of CRN.

		Definition
Na^+ currents	I_{Na}	Fast inward Na^+ current
	$I_{b,Na}$	Background Na^+ current
K^+ currents	I_{K1}	Inward rectifier K^+ current
	I_{Kur}	Ultrarapid delayed rectifier K^+ current
	I_{Kr}	Rapid delayed rectifier K^+ current
	I_{Ks}	Slow delayed rectifier K^+ current
	I_{Kto}	Transient outward K^+ current
Ca^{2+} currents	$I_{Ca,L}$	L-type inward Ca^{2+} current
	$I_{p,Ca}$	Outward Ca^{2+} pump current
	$I_{b,Ca}$	Background Ca^{2+} current
Mixed currents	$I_{Na,K}$	Na^+-K^+-pump current
	$I_{Na,Ca}$	Na^+-Ca^{2+}-exchanger current

Table 2.2: CRN Model constants [71].

	Definition	Value
C_m	Membrane capacitance	100 pF
V_{cell}	Cell volume	20 100 μm^3
V_i	Intracellular volume	13 668 μm^3
V_{up}	SR uptake compartment volume	1 109.52 μm^3
V_{rel}	SR release compartment volume	96.48 μm^3
$[K^+]_{out}$	Extracellular K^+ concentration	5.4 mM
$[Na^+]_{out}$	Extracellular Na^+ concentration	140 mM
$[Ca^{2+}]_{out}$	Extracellular Ca^{2+} concentration	1.8 mM

compartments (fig. 2.18). A more detailed description of the equations, parameters, constants, and quantitative values can be found in [71].

2.6 Bidomain Model

Excitation spread within the heart is based on myocytes coupled through gap junctions. In computer models of the heart this coupling of cardiac myocytes is represented by models of current flow in tissue. These models can reconstruct the current flowing through the intracellular and extracellular space.

The bidomain model is a mathematical model of the electrical properties of cardiac muscle cells, that takes into account the anisotropy of both the intracellular

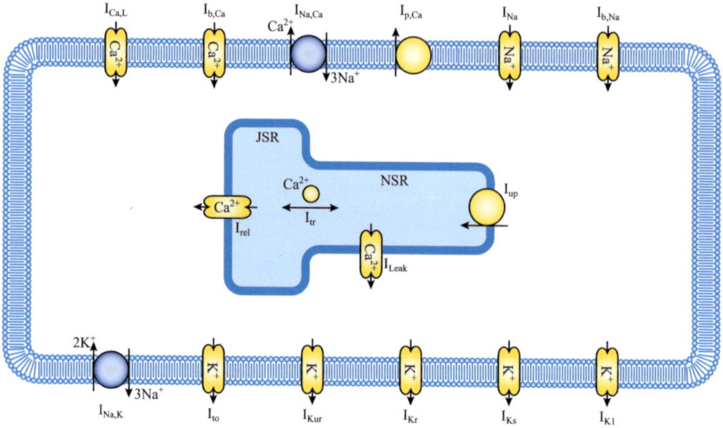

Fig. 2.18: A schematic representation of the Courtemanche-Ramirez-Nattel cell model with currents, pumps and exchangers included in the model (adapted from `www.cellml.org`).

and extracellular space. The intracellular and extracellular space can be modeled with different electrical conductivity in various directions and also the degree of anisotropy can be different in the two spaces. The two domains are separated by the cell membrane, through which the currents between the two domains flow. The bidomain model predicts the electrical behavior averaged over many cells. For each domain the distribution of electric potentials can be described with the Poisson's equation for stationary electrical field:

$$\nabla(\sigma_i \nabla \Phi_i) = \beta I_m - I_{si} \tag{2.8}$$

$$\nabla(\sigma_e \nabla \Phi_e) = -\beta I_m - I_{se}, \tag{2.9}$$

where Φ_i and Φ_e are the intracellular and extracellular potentials, respectively, σ_i and σ_e the corresponding volume-averaged conductivity tensors, I_m the transmembrane current density, β the surface to volume ratio of the cells, and I_{si} and I_{se} externally applied currents.

The two domains Φ_i and Φ_e are connected via the membrane voltage V_m.

$$V_m = \Phi_i - \Phi_e \tag{2.10}$$

If no external stimulus currents are applied, the equations can be reformulated to

$$\nabla((\sigma_i + \sigma_e)\nabla\Phi_e) = -\nabla(\sigma_i\nabla V_m). \tag{2.11}$$

This is the first part of the bidomain model. It describes how the transmembrane voltage V_m (calculated from an electrophysiological cell model) influences the extracellular potential. Inserting (2.10) into (2.9) leads to

$$\begin{aligned}\nabla(\sigma_i\nabla\Phi_i) &= \nabla(\sigma_i\nabla(V_m + \Phi_e)) \\ &= \nabla(\sigma_i\nabla V_m) + \nabla(\sigma_i\nabla\Phi_e) \\ &= \beta I_m - I_{si}.\end{aligned} \tag{2.12}$$

Inserting the ion current I_m (2.13) flowing through the membran into (2.12)

$$I_m = \beta_m(C_m\frac{dV}{dt} + I_m) \tag{2.13}$$

leads to

$$\nabla(\sigma_i\nabla V_m) + \nabla\cdot(\sigma_i\nabla\Phi_e) = \beta\cdot(C_m\frac{dV}{dt} + I_m) - I_{si}. \tag{2.14}$$

This is the second bidomain equation and describes the influence of the intracellular and extracellular current on the stimulus current, which in its turn serves as input for the cell models [72].

3

Mathematical & Signal Processing Fundamentals

In the following chapter the mathematical methods and signal processing methods used in this thesis are introduced.

3.1 Statistic Measures

A random process is described by a stochastic variable X. For this stochastic variable a distribution function $\mathrm{D}(x)$ is defined as

$$\mathrm{D}(x) := \mathrm{P}(X \leq x) \quad (3.1)$$

$$= \int_{-\infty}^{x} f(u)\, du, \quad (3.2)$$

with the probability P. The distribution function $\mathrm{D}(x)$ is related to a continuous probability density function $f(x)$ [73]. So, $f(x)$ (when existent) is the first derivative of the distribution function

$$f(x) = \mathrm{D}'(x). \quad (3.3)$$

Probability distributions can be described based on the probability density function (PDF). There are several characteristic values of a probability density that will be introduced hereafter.

3.1.1 Expectation Value

The expectation value or mean of a stochastic variable X is defined as the integral of the random variable with respect to its probability measure

$$\mathrm{E}\{X\} = \int_{-\infty}^{\infty} x \cdot f(x)\, dx = \mu_X. \tag{3.4}$$

3.1.2 Central Moments

To describe the spread, asymmetry, and curvature of a stochastic distribution higher moments are introduced [73]. The kth central moment is defined as

$$\mathrm{E}\{[X-\mathrm{E}\{X\}]^k\} = \int_{-\infty}^{\infty} [x-\mathrm{E}\{X\}]^k\, f(x)\, dx = \mu_X^k \tag{3.5}$$

The second central moment is called the variance $\mathrm{Var}(X)$. The variance is a measure of the spread of data. A large variance value indicates a large spread of the data around the mean.

$$\mathrm{Var}(X) = \mathrm{E}\{[X-\mathrm{E}\{X\}]^2\} = \sigma_X^2 \tag{3.6}$$

The standard deviation σ_X is the square root of the variance

$$\sigma_X = \sqrt{\mathrm{Var}(X)}. \tag{3.7}$$

The third central moment normalized to σ^3 is a measure of the asymmetry of a distribution. It is called skewness and defined as

$$\mathrm{Skew}(X) = \mathrm{E}\left\{\left[\frac{X-\mathrm{E}\{X\}}{\sigma}\right]^3\right\} = \frac{\mu_X^3}{\sigma_X^3}. \tag{3.8}$$

A negative skewness indicates that the tail on the left side of the PDF is longer than the tail on the right side and the bulk of the values lies to the right of the mean. A positive skewness indicates that the tail on the right side is longer than the one on the left side and the bulk of the values lies to the left of the mean. If the values are symmetrically distributed on both sides of the mean, the skewness is zero.
The fourth standardized moment (kurtosis) is a measure of the peakedness of a PDF.

$$\mathrm{Kurt}(X) = \mathrm{E}\left\{\left[\frac{X-\mathrm{E}\{X\}}{\sigma}\right]^4\right\} = \frac{\mu_X^4}{\sigma_X^4} \tag{3.9}$$

3.1.3 Covariance and Correlation

The correlation coefficient is a measure of the linear dependence of two stochastic variables or stochastic processes. To calculate the correlation coefficient first the covariance is introduced. The covariance for two stochastic variables X and Y is defined by the expectation value

$$\mathrm{Cov}(X,Y) = \mathrm{E}\left\{ \left[X - \mathrm{E}(X)\right]\left[Y - \mathrm{E}(Y)\right] \right\}. \tag{3.10}$$

Variance (eq. (3.6)) is a special case of covariance, where the two stochastic variables are similar.
Subsequently, Pearson's correlation coefficient ρ between two variables X and Y is defined as the covariance (Cov) of the two variables divided by the product of their standard deviations (σ):

$$\rho(X,Y) = \frac{\mathrm{Cov}(X,Y)}{\sigma_X \sigma_Y}, \qquad |\rho| \leq 1. \tag{3.11}$$

The correlation coefficient can be in the range between -1 and 1. $\rho = 1$ implies lineare dependence and $\rho = -1$ negative linear dependence. If $\rho = 0$ the two stochastic variables are linear independent.

3.1.4 Normal Distribution

Gaussian (normal) distributed stochastic variables play an important role in practical applications. Is the actual probability density function unknown, often a normal distribution is assumed [74].
Given is the stochastic variable X with expected value μ and variance σ^2. The stochastic variable X is normal distributed, when its probability density function is

$$f(x) = \frac{1}{\sqrt{2\pi\sigma^2}} \cdot \exp\left(-\frac{(x-\mu)^2}{2\sigma^2}\right). \tag{3.12}$$

A normal distribution with $\mu = 0$ and $\sigma^2 = 1$ is called standardized normal distribution.
The fourth standardized moment (kurtosis) is a measure of the similarity of a given probability density function and the normal distribution. The kurtosis of an arbitrary normal distribution is always 3. Therefore, the excess is defined as

$$\text{Excess}(X) = \text{Kurt}(X) - 3. \tag{3.13}$$

The excess of a normal distribution equals 0. The excess attains positive values for distributions that have a sharper peak and longer, more pronounced tails, while it attains negative values for distributions that have a more rounded peak and shorter tails.

3.1.5 Boxplot

A boxplot (box-whisker-plot) is a quick way of examining one or more sets of data graphically. The distribution of a data set is visualized by a box (represented by the median, the first (Q1) and the third quartile (Q3)) and the whiskers (indicating the range of the data). The range between first and third quartile is called interquartile range (IQR). 50% of all values will be found in the IQR. The ends of the whiskers can represent several possible alternative values [75, 76]. Here they are defined as $Q1 - 1.5 \cdot IQR$ and $Q3 + 1.5 \cdot IQR$ and mark the extreme value limits. Data points outside the whiskers are marked as outlier.

While comparing two or more data sets, a possibility to get a first impression of the statistical difference between their medians are notches. Notches offer a rough impression of significance of the difference of medians. If the notches of two boxes do not overlap, this implies a statistically significant difference between the medians on a 5% level.

Figure 3.1 depicts an example boxplot. In this example two classes and their feature values are compared. From the interpretation of these boxplots one can figure out if there is a valuable threshold to distinguish between these two classes on the given feature. Figure 3.2 shows the boxplot representation of a normal distribution compared to the probability density function of the same normal distribution.

3.2 Kernel Density Estimation

A shortcoming of the boxplot representation is, that boxplots will not reflect the maximum dispersion of multimodal distributions. To give a more accurate view on multimodal distributions kernel density estimation is used. Kernel density estimation is a non-parametric way to estimate the probability density function (PDF) of a random variable. It is closely related to the histogram, but can be endowed with properties such as smoothness or continuity. Kernel estimators centre a ker-

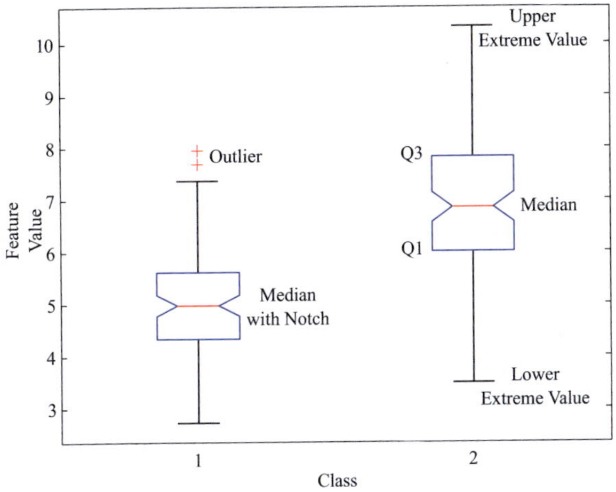

Fig. 3.1: Boxplot example of two different distributions. The box marks the first and third quartile. Notches around the median offer an impression of the difference between medians on a 5% level. Extreme values are marked by the whiskers and outliers by red crosses.

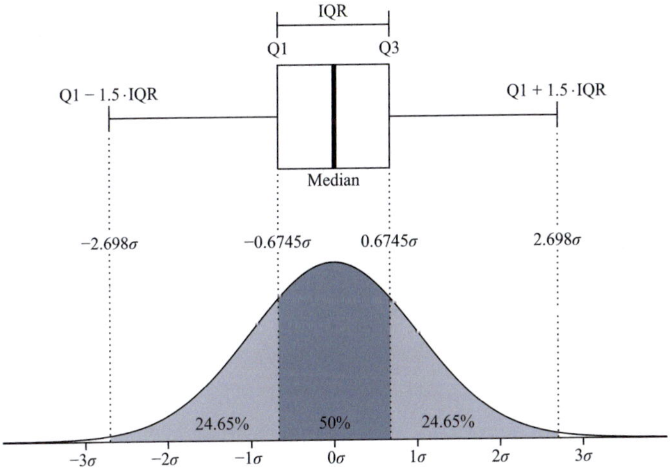

Fig. 3.2: Boxplot representation of a Gaussian (normal) distribution and its probability density function.

nel function at each data point x. The kernels are summed to make the kernel density estimate.

$$\hat{P}_h(x) = \frac{1}{nh} \sum_{i=1}^{n} K\left(\frac{x - x_i}{h}\right), \tag{3.14}$$

where K is the kernel and $h > 0$ is a smoothing parameter. The width of the kernels is given by h. Commonly used kernel functions are: Gaussian, triangular, box, biweight, Epanechnikov, and others [77].

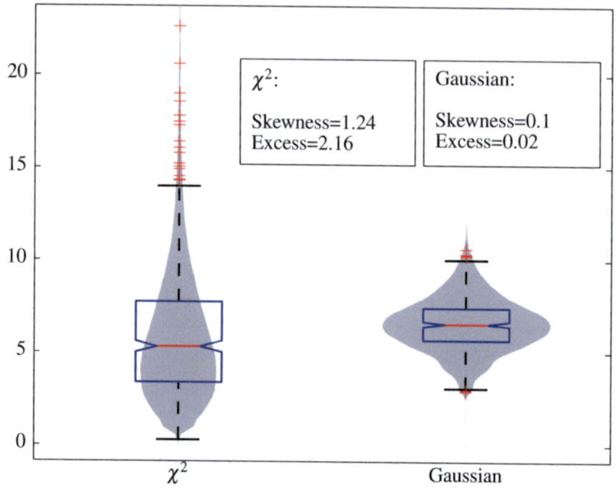

Fig. 3.3: Comparison of boxplots of χ^2-distributed and Gaussian (normal) distributed data. In addition to the boxplots the kernel density function of the distributions is depicted. The deviation of skewness and excess values is due to a finite number of samples.

Choosing h is crucial in density estimation. A large h will over-smooth the estimation and mask the structure of the data, whereas a small h will yield an estimation that is spiky and hard to interpret. The value of h in this work is based on a robust estimate of the standard deviation of the data and the kernel is chosen as Gaussian normal [77].

Figure 3.3 depicts a combined view of boxplot representation and PDF estimation for a χ^2 distribution and a Gaussian distribution. Together with the excess and the skewness, an unknown distribution of a data set can be described.

3.3 Entropy

Shannon's entropy H is a measure for the expectation value of the information contained in a message. In the context of information theory, a "message" is a specific realization of a random variable X [78]. That means, the entropy measures the average information content of a source with the character content $X = x_1, x_2, \ldots, x_N$.

$$\mathrm{H}(X) = -\sum_{i=1}^{N} p_i \cdot \mathrm{ld}(p_i) \text{ bit} \tag{3.15}$$

p_i denotes the probability of occurrence of x_i. In the context of signal processing the entropy is also used as a measure of the degree of organization of a signal. Shannon's entropy has maximum values, if the signal's development over time is not predictable.

3.4 Analytic Signal & Hilbert Transformation

An analytic signal has only spectral components at positive frequencies [79]. A regular way to produce an analytical signal of a real-valued signal $x(t)$ is to add an imaginary part that is identical to the Hilbert transform $\mathcal{H}$ of $x(t)$.

$$z(t) = x(t) + j \cdot \mathcal{H}[x(t)] \tag{3.16}$$

The Hilbert-Transformation produces a real-valued signal, that has shifted frequency components. It has the effect of shifting the phase of the negative frequency components of $x(t)$ by +90° and the phase of the positive frequency components by –90°. The Hilbert-Transformation is defined by the use of the quadrature filter with the impulse response $g_Q(t)$ and the frequency response $G_Q(f)$ [80]:

$$g_Q(t) = \begin{cases} 1/\pi t & ,t \neq 0 \\ 0 & ,t = 0 \end{cases} \qquad G_Q(f) = \begin{cases} -j & ,f > 0 \\ 0 & ,f = 0 \\ j & ,f < 0 \end{cases} \tag{3.17}$$

The magnitude of the analytic signal $z(t)$ is the complex envelope of the original signal $x(t)$.

3.5 Fourier Transform

The frequency content of a periodic function can be analyzed with the Fourier series (eq. (3.18)). Periodic functions are decomposed into trigonometric functions (Fourier analysis). The periodic function $f(t)$ is represented by an infinite sum of sines and cosines. The result of this decomposition is an infinite number of harmonic frequencies and their amplitudes. By the use of these harmonics the periodic function can be composed.

$$f(t) = \frac{a_0}{2} + \sum_{k=1}^{\infty} \left(a_k \cos(2\pi \frac{k}{T} t) + b_k \sin(2\pi \frac{k}{T} t) \right) \tag{3.18}$$

T is the cycle duration of $f(t)$, a_k and b_k are named Fourier coefficients. Another definition of the Fourier series is the exponential definition of (3.18)

$$f(t) = \sum_{-\infty}^{+\infty} \underline{c}_n e^{jn\omega t} \quad \text{with} \quad \underline{c}_n = \frac{1}{T} \int_0^T f(t) e^{-jn\omega t} dt, \tag{3.19}$$

where $\underline{c}_n$ is the complexe amplitude of $f(t)$.

3.5.1 Continuous Fourier Transform

To analyze also non-periodic signals the cycle duration is set to $T \to \infty$. This leads from Fourier series to the Fourier integral [81]. Therefore the limit

$$\lim_{T \to \infty} (\underline{c}_n T) = F(j\omega) \tag{3.20}$$

is build. This limit is named spectral density. With $\omega = 2\pi f$ follows

$$\begin{aligned} f(t) &\circ\!\!-\!\!\bullet F(f) \\ F(f) &= \int_{-\infty}^{\infty} f(t) e^{-j2\pi f t} dt. \end{aligned} \tag{3.21}$$

From the exponential definition (3.19) follows the inverse Fourier transform

$$\begin{aligned} F(f) &\bullet\!\!-\!\!\circ f(t) \\ f(t) &= \int_{-\infty}^{\infty} F(f) e^{j2\pi f t} df. \end{aligned} \tag{3.22}$$

The absolute value of the Fourier Transform $|F(f)|$ is denoted as frequency spectrum of $f(t)$. The spectrum corresponds to the energy of the particular frequency components in the signal.

3.5.2 Discrete Fourier Transform and Fast Fourier Transform

To analyse continuous signals with help of digital computers the signal as well as its spectrum must be discrete. The signal $x(t)$ is discretized with sampling frequency f_A and sampling time $T_A = 1/f_A$, respectively. x_k is the time-discrete representation of the continuous signal $x(t)$ [82, 83],

$$x(t)|_{t=kT_A} = x(kT_A) =: x_k, \tag{3.23}$$

k is an integer within the range $-\infty < k < +\infty$. As only a finite number N of sample values is reasonable, k is applicatory in the range of $0 < k < N-1$. The discrete Fourier transform (DFT) and the inverse discrete Fourier transform (IDFT) are defined as [82, 83]

$$\begin{aligned} X_n = \mathrm{DFT}\{x_k\} &= \sum_{k=0}^{N-1} x_k e^{-j2\pi kn/N} \\ x_k = \mathrm{IDFT}\{X_n\} &= \frac{1}{N}\sum_{n=0}^{N-1} X_n e^{j2\pi kn/N}. \end{aligned} \tag{3.24}$$

The computational complexity of the DFT is $O(N^2)$ and is directly dependent to the signal's length N. Using symmetry and periodicity in the DFT algorithm, the computational costs can be reduced to $N\log(N)$ [82, 83]. The family of algorithms that are more efficient than the DFT are denoted fast Fourier transform (FFT) algorithms.

3.5.3 Short Time Fourier Transform

The Fourier transform gives information about the frequency content of a signal. But, it can not give an information at which time a frequency has occurred. The short time Fourier transform (STFT) provides this information and is a method to analyze also non-stationary signals. Therefore, only short periods of the signal are Fourier transformed. The signal $f(t)$ is multiplied with a window function $w(t)$ that is non-zero for a short period of time and only this non-zero part is transformed into the frequency domain. Thus, the signal is transformed into the time-frequency domain [79]

$$S(w,t) = \int_{-\infty}^{\infty} s(\tau)\, w(\tau - t)\, e^{-jw\tau} d\tau. \tag{3.25}$$

The quality of the STFT is strongly dependent on the window function w. In addition the resolutions of time and frequency in the time-frequency domain are inversely proportional.

$$\Delta w \cdot \Delta t \leqslant \frac{1}{2} \tag{3.26}$$

A narrow window function results in a poor frequency resolution, whereas a broad window function results in better frequency resolution but less time domain resolution [79].

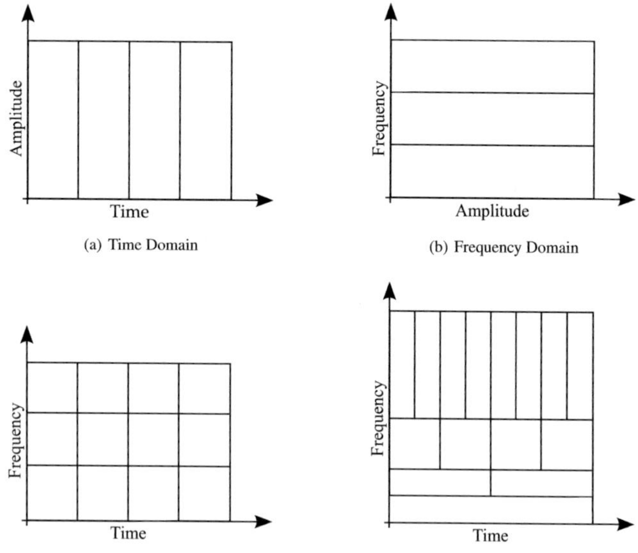

(a) Time Domain

(b) Frequency Domain

(c) Time-Frequency Domain, STFT

(d) Time-Frequency Domain, WT

Fig. 3.4: Comparison between time, frequency, and time-frequency domain representations.

3.6 Wavelet Transformation

The Fourier and wavelet transforms (WT) measure similarity between a signal and an analyzing function (kernel function). Both transforms use the inner product as this measure of similarity, but differ in their choice of analyzing functions. The Fourier transform uses complex exponentials, whereas the so called wavelets are used by the wavelet transform. The wavelet transform is a time-frequency transformation. A signal is transposed into the time-frequency domain by the WT. Compared to the FFT, the WT gives not only information about the frequency content of a signal, but also information at which time segment a frequency occurs. A signal is represented in different time-frequency segments with different time-frequency scales (fig. 3.4). The continuous wavelet transform is defined as

$$W_x^{\Psi}(a,b;f(t),\psi(t)) = \frac{1}{\sqrt{|a|}} \int_{-\infty}^{\infty} x(t)\psi^* \left(\frac{t-b}{a}\right) dt. \tag{3.27}$$

The kernel function of the WT is a wavelet $\psi(t)$. A wavelet is a continuous, zero-mean energy signal that fulfills the requirement

$$\int_{-\infty}^{+\infty} \frac{|\Psi(af)|^2}{|f|} df < \infty, \tag{3.28}$$

with Fourier transform $\Psi(f)$ of $\psi(t)$. The function $\psi(t)$ is also called mother wavelet. Figure 3.5 shows three different often used wavelets. The Haar wavelet is a simple wavelet that is often used to find zero crossings in a signal. In this work Daubechie's wavelet of order 11 is used to remove baseline wander from a signal (sec. 4.4.1). Coiflet 4 is used for analyzing the fractionation of atrial electrograms (sec. 7.7). The mother wavelet is scaled by a and time shifted with b to compute the WT. To ensure that the wavelet $\psi_{a,b}(t)$ is not changing its signal energy while scaling, the scaling function is adjusted with $1/\sqrt{|a|}$.

$$\psi_{a,b}(t) = \frac{1}{\sqrt{|a|}} \psi \left(\frac{t-b}{a}\right). \tag{3.29}$$

As result of the scaling function time duration and bandwidth are changed in dependence of the mean time-shift and frequency-shift.

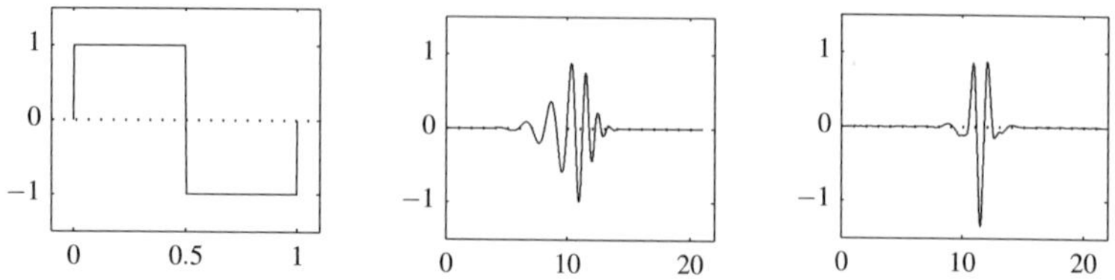

(a) Haar Wavelet (b) Daubechies D11 (c) Coiflet 4

Fig. 3.5: Three examples of frequently used wavelets.

3.6.1 Discrete Wavelet Transformation

Corresponding to the discrete Fourier transform the discrete wavelet transform (DWT) must be defined to use the WT with digital systems. Therefore, the scaling factor a as well as the shifting parameter b must be discretized. a and b are chosen to $a = a_0^m$ and $b = k b_0 a_0^m$, where $m,n \in \mathbb{Z}$ range over Z, and $a_0 > 1$ and $b_0 > 0$ are fixed [84]. This corresponds to the discrete representation of a wavelet family

$$\psi_{m,n}(kT_A) = {a_0}^{-m/2} \psi\left(\frac{kT_A - k b_0 a_0^m}{a_0^m}\right), \tag{3.30}$$

with the time discretization kT_A (sec. 3.5.2).

Wavelet Filter Bank

One way to realize a discrete wavelet transform is by use of filters. Compared to the WT, which is a correlation between a wavelet at different scales and the signal with the scale (or the frequency) being used as a measure of similarity, the DWT represents the same information, but discretized. The WT is computed by changing the scale of the analysis window, shifting the window in time, multiplying by the signal, and integrating over all times. In the discrete case, filters with different cutoff frequencies are used to analyze the signal at different scales. Therefore, the signal is passed through a series of high pass filters to analyze the high frequency parts (details) and it is passed through a series of low pass filters to analyze the low frequency parts (approximations).

$$
\begin{aligned}
y_{high}(n) &= \sum_{k=-\infty}^{\infty} x(k)h(2n-k) \\
y_{low}(n) &= \sum_{k=-\infty}^{\infty} x(k)g(2n-k)
\end{aligned} \tag{3.31}
$$

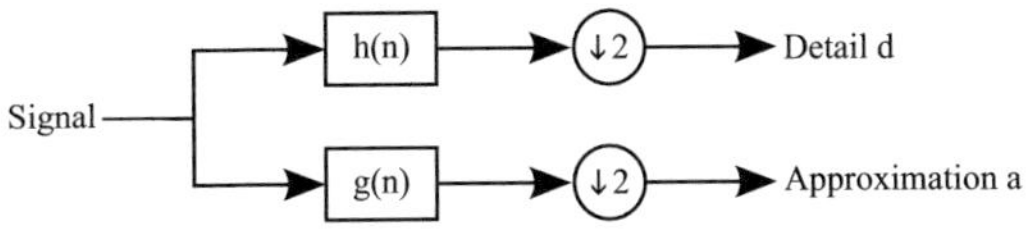

Fig. 3.6: Block diagram of the wavelet filterbank analysis principle. The high-pass filter is characterized by its impulse response h, the low-pass filter by its impulse response g. After the filtering the resulting signal is downsampled by 2.

The filters are characterized by their impulse responses h and g (3.6). The signal is decomposed using a high-pass filter h and a low-pass filter g simultaneously n times according to the detail or approximation level that should be reached. At each level the two filters are related to each other and since half of the frequencies of the signal are removed by the filters at each level, half of the samples can be discarded according to the Shannon-Nyquist theorem [85, 86]. Hence, the filter outputs are subsampled by 2. Figure 3.7 depicts an implementation of a wavelet filterbank down to level 3. Outputs of the filterbank are the detail coefficients for each level and the approximation details for the 3rd level [87].

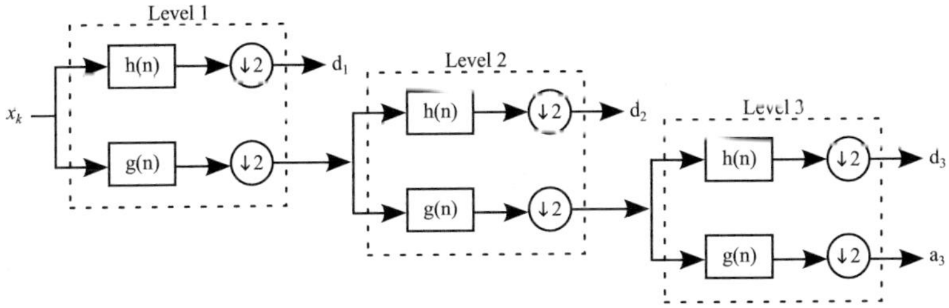

Fig. 3.7: A 3-level wavelet filterbank. Assuming the highest frequency component of x_k is 1024 Hz, d_1 represents the frequency band 513 – 1024 Hz, d_2 the frequency band 257 – 512 Hz, d_3 the frequency band 129 – 256 Hz, and a_3 the frequency band 0 – 128 Hz.

3.7 Principle Component Analysis

Principle Component Analysis (PCA) is a classical tool in statistical data analysis to reduce the number of variables or to detect structure in the relationship between variables, that is to classify variables. Therefore, PCA is applied as a data reduction or structure detection method. The PCA transforms a number of correlated variables into a smaller number of uncorrelated variables (principle components, PCs), preserving all or most of the information. The first principal component covers as much of the variability in the data as possible, and each succeeding component covers as much of the remaining variability as possible. This is done by finding an orthonormal base that transforms the data into a subspace with decreasing covariances over the axes (fig. 3.8).

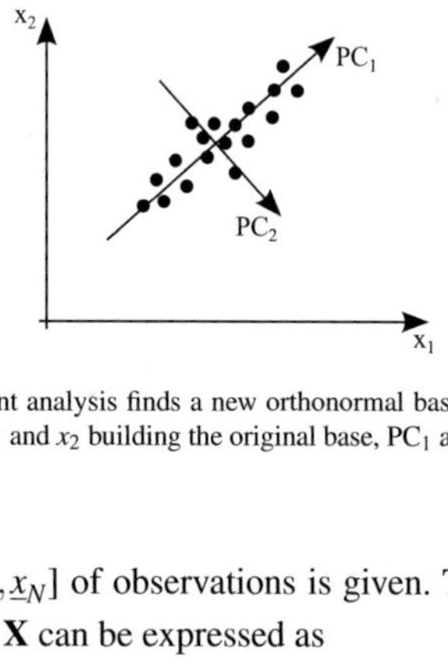

Fig. 3.8: The principle component analysis finds a new orthonormal base so that the variances along the new axes is maximal. x_1 and x_2 building the original base, PC_1 and PC_2 are the axes found by the PCA.

A sample $\mathbf{X} = [\underline{x}_0, \underline{x}_1, \ldots, \underline{x}_N]$ of observations is given. The aim of the PCA is to find a new base $\mathbf{A}$ so that $\mathbf{X}$ can be expressed as

$$\mathbf{X} = \mathbf{Z}\mathbf{A}^{\mathrm{T}}. \tag{3.32}$$

The solution of the problem above is given by the eigenvalue decomposition of the observation covariance matrix $\mathbf{R}$ of the zero-mean data matrix $\mathbf{X}_{\mathrm{Z}}$:

$$\mathbf{R} = \mathbf{X}_{\mathrm{Z}}^{\mathrm{T}}\mathbf{X}_{\mathrm{Z}}. \tag{3.33}$$

The mean is subtracted from the data $\mathbf{X}$ to set the point of origin into the center of gravity of the data. Now only the variations from the mean will be examined. In which way the axes must be rotated to achieve the minimum covariance between the sample points is given by the covariance matrix **R**. The covariance matrix is a square matrix. The principal diagonale of this matrix is filled with variance values, whereas the rest of the matrix is filled with covariances. If this matrix is diagonalized only the variances of the diagonalized coordinates are remaining and these coordinates will give the directions (loadings) of the new axes [88, 89]. Any square, symmetric, nonsingular matrix can be transformed to a diagonal matrix using

$$\mathbf{L} = \mathbf{A}^{\mathrm{T}}\mathbf{R}\mathbf{A}, \tag{3.34}$$

where the columns of **A** contain the eigenvectors of **R**, and **L** is a diagonal matrix with the eigenvalues along the diagonal [90]. The eigenvalues are ordered descending $\lambda_1 \geq \lambda_2 \geq \ldots \geq \lambda_N$, with the same order imposed on the corresponding eigenvectors. The eigenvectors of **R** are used to obtain new variables called principal components (PCs). The diagonal elements (eigenvalues) of **L** are the variances of the new data. The eigenvalues of the covariance matrix **R** correspond to the variances of the rotated variables (principle components). The PCA solution is given by

$$\mathbf{Z}_{PCA} = \mathbf{X}_z\mathbf{A} \tag{3.35}$$

Z contains the principal component scores (transformed data) and **A** contains the eigenvectors of **R** which will give the base of the new coordinate system (PCs=transformed variables).

3.8 Decision Trees

A method or an algorithm that divides objects into different classes is called classifier. A classifier uses parametric or non-parametric attributes (features, descriptors) of these objects to assign them to classes. A classifier assigns new observations with unknown class belonging to a class based on explicit rules or a given training data set containing observations with known class membership. Automatic classification systems are used in artificial intelligence, pattern recognition, computer vision, document classification, etc. There are a lot of different classification algorithms. The most used classifiers are the neural network (multi-layer perceptron), support vector machines, distance measures in a n-dimensional feature space, Gaussian mixture model, naive Bayes, and decision trees.

In this work a decision tree is used as classifier. Amongst other data mining methods, decision trees have three main advantages. First, a decision tree is easy to understand and easy to interpret [91]. They use a so called white box model. If a given situation is observable in a model the explanation for the condition is explained by boolean logic. In contrast, artificial neural networks e.g. are an example of a black box model. It is not obvious what is happening in hidden layers. Second, decision trees require little data preparation and are able to handle both numerical and categorical data. Other techniques often require data normalization, removal of blank values, and dummy variables need to be created. Third, it is possible to validate a tree using statistical tests. So, the reliability of a decision tree can be calculated. Finally, decision trees are robust decision makers even if its assumptions are violated by the true model from which the data was generated [92,93] and they can be used on multi-class problems [91].

A decision or classification tree represents a multi-stage decision process. The complexity and semantic of the decision rules are not limited. For binary decision trees each rule term can attain only one out of two values. At each stage a binary decision is made. A tree is composed of nodes and branches. The nodes are divided into one root node, any number of inner nodes, and at least two terminal nodes (leafs). Inner nodes split into two children, while terminal nodes do not have any children. Each inner node represents a logical rule and each leaf an answer to the decision problem. Regularly, these answers are class labels. Each observation that falls into a particular leaf is assigned to that class. A simple example tree is depicted in figure 3.9. The root node is represented by n_1, the inner nodes by $n_2 - n_4$, and the leaf nodes by $L_1 - L_5$.

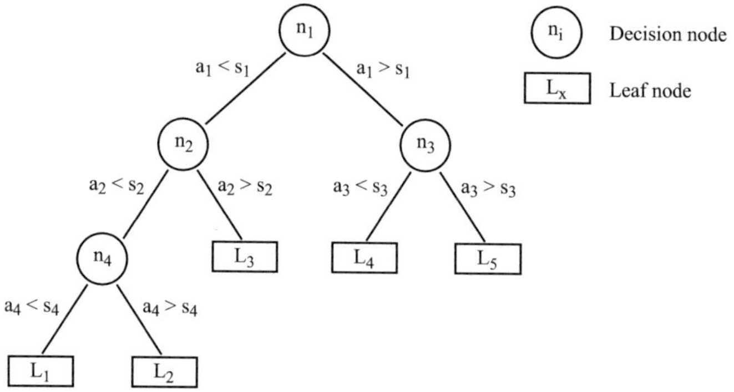

Fig. 3.9: Schematic diagram of a binary decision tree. At each node n_i a given attribute a_k is compared to the split value s_l and the according path is chosen.

3.8.1 Tree Induction

The idea behind a decision tree is to split the n-dimensional attribute (feature) space into partitions, such that the majority of members of one partition belong to one class. The induction (growing) of a decision tree is done top-down. A data set with reliable experience values to the decision problem is crucial (training data set). This means the classification for each object of the training data set must be known. At each node the attribute is searched that splits the training data set most effectively according to the given classes. Entropy, Information-Gain-Ratio [94], or Gini-Diversity-Index [91] can be used as measure for the best classification. The found attribute then is used to split the data set into subsets. This procedure is done recursively on the resulting subsets until there is only one class per subset remaining or a stop criterion is reached [95].
Algorithms for automatic tree induction all use the recursive top-down principle, but they use different methods to choose the best attribute to split the data, to stop the growth, and to optimize the resulting tree. The two main algorithms are the CART-algorithm (Classification And Regression Tree) [91] and the C 4.5-algorithm [94] which extends the ID3-algorithm (Iterative Dichotomiser 3) [96]. Another popular algorithm is the SLIQ (Supervised Learning In Quest) which is a computation time optimizing version of the CART algorithm [97].
The induction process can be described in a simplified way by

1. set root node
2. choose attribute and split point for most significant split
3. split data
4. repeat step 2 – 3 until all objects are assigned or a stop criterion is reached.

3.8.2 Splitting Criteria

Splitting the data at a node should result in an increasing relative membership of one class in the child nodes. That implies that after a split, the purity of classes is rising. To find the best attribute a_k to split the training data ω at a node n_i, Information-Gain-Ratio (IGR) and Gini-Diversity-Index (GDI) are the most common used algorithms. IGR is used by the C4.5 algorithm introduced by Quinlan [94] and GDI is the standard algorithm used by Breiman for the CART algorithm [91]. Both criterions are measures for the purity of classes after a split.

3.8.2.1 Information Gain Ratio

C4.5 uses information gain as its attribute selection measure. It is based on Shannon's entropy H (sec. 3.3). The entropy of a given training data set ω which is divided into M classes is given by

$$\mathrm{H}(\omega) = -\sum_{m=1}^{M} p_m \cdot \mathrm{ld}\,(p_m), \tag{3.36}$$

with p_m the probability of the occurrence of objects with class membership m. The information gain (IG) is the reduction of the entropy caused by splitting the training data ω at node n_i [98]

$$\mathrm{IG}(n_i, a_k(s_l)) = \mathrm{H}(\omega) - \sum_{c=1}^{C} \frac{|\omega_c|}{|\omega|} \cdot \mathrm{H}(\omega_c), \tag{3.37}$$

where s_l is the used split point on attribute a_k. C is the number of a node's children. For a binary tree C equals 2. The cardinality of the objects assigned to the node's children is $|\omega_c|$ and $|\omega|$ is the cardinality of the objects ω. IG is computed to estimate the gain produced by a split over an attribute, but IG tends to favor attributes that have a large number of values. To compensate for this Quinlan [99] suggests using information gain ratio instead of IG. Therefore, the split information (SI) is introduced:

$$\mathrm{SI}(n_i, a_k(s_l)) = -\sum_{c=1}^{C} \frac{|\omega_c|}{|\omega|} \cdot \mathrm{ld}\left(\frac{|\omega_c|}{|\omega|}\right). \tag{3.38}$$

SI is the information due to the split of ω on the basis of the value of the attribute a_k. The quotient of IG and SI yields the Information-Gain-Ratio (IGR)

$$\mathrm{IGR}(n_i, a_k(s_l)) = \frac{IG(n_i, a_k(s_l))}{SI(n_i, a_k(s_l))}. \tag{3.39}$$

3.8.2.2 Gini-Diversity-Index

The Gini-Diversity-Index (GDI) is used by Breiman's CART algorithm [91]. The GDI is used to measure the purity of possible child nodes, with the aim of maximizing the average purity of two child nodes when splitting. The GDI considers a binary split for each attribute and is defined as

$$\mathrm{GDI}(n_i) = 1 - \sum_{m=1}^{M} p^2(\omega_m|n_i). \tag{3.40}$$

This means an impurity function based on the GDI assigns an example to a class ω_m with the probability $p(m|t)$ in a node n_i. Finding the best split point at a node n_i is a two-step process. First, the best split point is searched for each attribute. Therefore, the attribute values of one attribute a_k are ordered according to size, starting with the smallest value

$$a_{kn} = (a_{k1}, a_{k2}, \ldots, a_{kp}) \quad \text{with} \quad a_{k1} < a_{k2} < \ldots < a_{kp}. \tag{3.41}$$

A reasonable split point s_l must lie between two attribute values and is defined as the arithmetic mean between two adjacent values a_p and a_{p+1}

$$s_{l,n} = a_{kn} + \frac{(a_{kn} - a_{kn+1})}{2}. \tag{3.42}$$

For each possible split point in the attribute value list the GDI is calculated and the split with the smallest GDI is chosen as best split point for this attribute. This procedure is repeated for each attribute. Second, the best attribute is searched that maximizes the reduction in impurity (minimal GDI) by a split.

3.8.3 Optimizing a Tree

Up to now, methods have been introduced to find the best possible split point at a particular node. Equally important is to determine the optimal tree size. Without any stop criterion the tree would grow until each leaf would represent only one object of the training data. As result this tree would fit best on the training data and the correct rate would be perfect. But using this over-specified tree on unknown data will result in significantly decreasing correct rates [95]. To stop the tree growing, respectively to stop the splitting process, a criterion is needed. A possible criterion is the change of the GDI, ΔGDI. If the purity does not increase by an additional split, this node will be defined as leaf node.

Applying a stop criterion during the induction process appeared not to be optimal [91]. As consequence the stop criterion is defined weak to get an oversized tree and do an optimization in a subsequent step. This leads to optimum tree size as well as better results [91]. Pruning is a technique that reduces the size of decision trees by removing sections of the tree that provide little power to classify instances.

Pruning should reduce the size of a decision tree without reducing predictive accuracy. In the following section Cost-Complexity-Pruning will be introduced as pruning method.

3.8.3.1 Cost-Complexity-Pruning

Cost-Complexity-Pruning (CCP) generates a series of trees starting with the maximal tree $T_{\max}$ and subsequently removing subtrees and substitute them with leaf nodes. At each step the resulting tree is evaluated with a cost function. This is done until all nodes are removed and only the root node T_0 is remaining. At the end all resulting trees will be compared according to their cost function value and the best tree will be chosen.

CCP uses a cost function including the classification error rate $R(T)$ as well as the number of used nodes. The cost-complexity measure $R_\alpha(T)$ is defined as a linear combination of the cost $R(T)$ of the tree and its complexity. The measure of the complexity of a tree is the total number of leaf nodes $|\tilde{T}|$ weighted with the continuous parameter α ($\alpha \in \mathbb{R}, \alpha \geq 0$).

$$R_\alpha(T) = R(T) + \alpha|\tilde{T}| \tag{3.43}$$

The tree's error rate is defined as the sum over all error rates of its leaf nodes:

$$R(T) = \sum_{t \in \tilde{T}} R(t). \tag{3.44}$$

Aim of the algorithm is to find a sequence of trees so that each subsequent tree is smaller than its preceding tree, $T_i > T_{i+1}$. CCP works by weakest-link cutting [91]. That implies that the error rate $R(T)$ of a node is always greater or equal than the error rate of the branch $R(T_t)$ originating from t. In other words, the classification rate is slightly increasing due to a split at node t. The costs for using a node t as a leaf node is the error rate plus the cost of a leaf node α

$$R_\alpha(t) = R(t) + \alpha \tag{3.45}$$

and the costs for a whole branch T_t are

$$R_\alpha(T_t) = R(T_t) + \alpha|\tilde{T}_t|, \tag{3.46}$$

with $R(T_t)$ the sum of error rates of the leaf nodes T_t.
For each value of α the subtree $T(\alpha) \leq T_{\max}$ is searched, that minimizes $R_\alpha(T)$. That means, if the error rate of a branch is greater or equal than the error rate of their preceding node, then this branch is pruned. As the penalty α per leaf node increases, the minimizing subtrees $T(\alpha)$ will have fewer leaf nodes [91]. As long as

$$R_\alpha(T_t) < R_\alpha(t), \tag{3.47}$$

the branch T_t has a smaller cost-complexity than the single node t. At a critical value of α the cost-complexities become equal and the subbranch is preferable. By inserting the cost functions into (3.47) the critical value for α can be derived

$$\alpha < \frac{R(t) - R(T_t)}{|\tilde{T}| - 1}. \tag{3.48}$$

Now, for the tree of step k the following function can be defined

$$g_k(t) = \begin{cases} \frac{R(t)-R(T_t)}{|\tilde{T}|-1}, t \notin \tilde{T}_k \\ +\infty, t \in \tilde{T}_k \end{cases} \tag{3.49}$$

and the weakest link can be found with

$$g_k(\bar{t_k}) = \min\{g_k(t)\}, t \in T_k. \tag{3.50}$$

The weakest link is at node t_k at which the subtree $T_{\bar{t_k}}$ is pruned from T_k. Thus, the tree of the next step T_{k+1} is reached and α_{k+1} is set to $g_k(\bar{t_k})$. The pruning is repeated until only the root node is left.

3.8.3.2 Cross Validation

To find the best tree that can be derived from the sample data and to evaluate how well a decision tree is going to perform on unknown data, there are two established approaches that estimate the error rate $\hat{R}(T_k)$. One way to estimate the predictive ability of a decision tree is to test it on a set of data not used in training but with "perfect" knowledge about the class of every member. The sample data is divided into a test set and a training set. A tree is built from the training set and the error rate is calculated with the "unknown" test set. However, often there is not enough data to allow a sufficient amount of data to be kept back for testing [100].

A more sophisticated version of evaluating a decision tree is the cross validation. For a cross validation the data set is divided randomly into V even subsets. One of the V subsets is used as test set and the other $V-1$ subsets are put together to form a training set. For each test set the error rate is computed and the average error across all V trials is calculated. The disadvantage of this method is that the training algorithm has to be rerun from scratch V times, which means it takes V times as much computation to make an evaluation [95, 100]. Breiman showed that dividing the sample data into $V = 10$ partitions is sufficient and using finer partitions does not significantly improve the result [91]. Breiman suggests in the CART algorithm that the best tree from the sequence of trees T_k is the tree T_k that has ideal size. As the trees in the sequence T_k are from different size and have different attributes and split points, they are classified by the weighting factor α. A tree T_k minimizes the cost function $R_\alpha(T)$ for all values $\alpha \in [\alpha_k, \alpha_{k+1}[$. T_{k+1} will be chosen for values $\geq \alpha_{k+1}$. To make a categorization a progression α'_k is defined by

$$\alpha'_k = \sqrt{\alpha_k \cdot \alpha_{k+1}}. \tag{3.51}$$

To each value α'_k a tree T_k^v from the cross validation sequence T_k^v will be assigned that fullfils

$$\alpha'_k \in [\,\alpha_k^{(v)}, \alpha_{k+1}^{(v)}\,[\,. \tag{3.52}$$

For the resulting categorization a new estimation $\hat{R}_{\alpha'_k}$ is gained as the mean of error rates $R(T_k^v)$ of trees assigned to α'_k. Breiman [91] showed that an optimal tree with minimal error rate exists. But it is difficult to determine this optimal tree from the estimation due to the spread of estimation results. Therefore, the tree is chosen as best fit that holds true for

$$\hat{R}(T_{\alpha'_k}) < \min(R(T_{\alpha'_k})) + \sigma(\min \hat{R}(T_{\alpha'_k})), \tag{3.53}$$

with $\sigma(\hat{R}_{T_k})$ is the standard deviation of error rates and N_T the number of test objects.

$$\sigma(\hat{R}_{T_k}) = \sqrt{\frac{\hat{R}_{T_k}(1-\hat{R}_{T_k})}{N_T}} \tag{3.54}$$

3.8.4 Class Membership of Leaf Nodes

The class affiliation of a leaf node is defined by the relative number of training objects in a node. The number of objects per node n_i is given by N_{n_i}. N_{n_i,ω_m} is the number of objects per class ω_m of this node.

$$p(\omega_m|n_i) = \frac{N_{n_i,\omega_m}}{N_{n_i}} \tag{3.55}$$

The conditional probability $p(\omega_m|n_i)$ computes the probability that an object at node n_i belongs to class ω_m [100]. The leaf node is assigned with the class membership of the highest probability $p(\omega_m|n_i)$. The error probability of a leaf node is

$$r(n_i) = 1 - \max\{p(\omega_m|n_i)\}. \tag{3.56}$$

With the definition of the probability that an object is assigned to node n_i

$$p(n_i) = \frac{N_{n_i}}{N} \tag{3.57}$$

follows the error rate $R(n_i)$ for this node n_i

$$R(n_i) = p(n_i)r(n_i). \tag{3.58}$$

Part II

Quantitative Analysis of Atrial Electrograms

4

Introduction and Preprocessing of Atrial Electrograms

4.1 Intra-atrial Electrograms

Intra-atrial electrograms are electric signals measured within the atria. Therefore, a catheter assembled with electrodes (fig. 2.13) is pushed via the iliac vein or the subclavian vein into the vena cava and finally into the right atrium. To measure signals within the left atrium, the catheter is pushed through the interatrial septum into the left atrium by puncturing. While touching the endocardium a potential difference between two electrodes can be measured. Once the catheter is placed, it can be used to record electrical activity (fig. 4.1). The two traditional methods for recording electrical signals are "unipolar" and "bipolar". In unipolar recoding only one catheter electrode is used, with the second electrode being located "far away". This electrode can be a surface electrode or Wilson's central terminal, which uses the mean of the extremity electrodes.
In the electrophysiology (EP) lab, bipolar recordings are most commonly used. To obtain bipolar signals, both measurement electrodes are placed on the catheter within the heart. Regularly neighboring electrodes are used. Bipolar recordings reflect the electrical activity of an area of tissue between the two electrodes by measuring the electrical near-field. Unipolar recordings give information about the electrical activity of the tissue directly beneath the electrode. Figure 4.2 depicts examples of unipolar and bipolar electrograms recorded in the coronary sinus. Additionally the surface ECG is shown. The atrial signals are tainted with ventricular activity. It can be seen, that ventricular activity in the bipolar recording is not as dominant as in the unipolar.

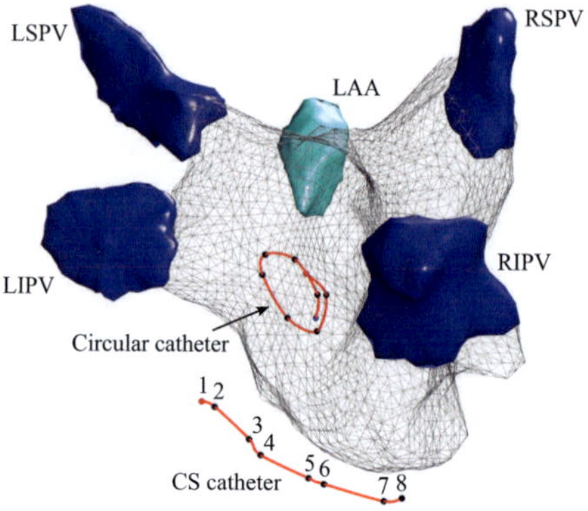

Fig. 4.1: Left atrial anatomy with commonly used catheters during an EP examination.

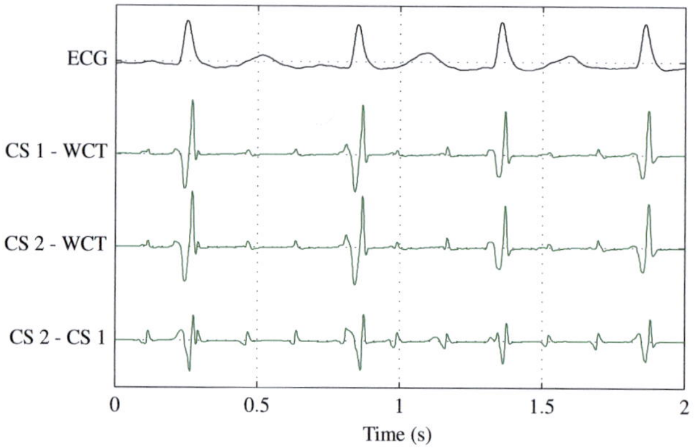

Fig. 4.2: Comparison of unipolar and bipolar signals. The catheter is placed within the coronary sinus and unipolar signals from electrode 1 and electrode 2, using WCT as indifferent electrode, are recorded. The bipolar electrogram is the potential difference between electrode 1 and 2. ECG lead I is shown as reference. All electrograms are tainted with ventricular far fields.

4.2 Complex Fractionated Atrial Electrograms (CFAEs)

Although there is consensus about the ablation strategy of paroxysmal AF, strategies for ablation of persistent AF are discussed controversially [46,101]. After isolating the pulmonary veins physicians search commonly for CFAEs that "mark"

the substrate maintaining AF. These signals are fractionated with different length and characteristics. Ablating CFAEs seems to be a promising method to terminate AF [101]. Therefore, understanding and interpretation of these CFAEs plays an important role. As shown by Konings [58] there are different types of fractionated electrograms during AF. Nademanee [102] defined CFAEs as:
Atrial electrograms

1. "that have fractionated electrograms composed of two deflections or more, and/or perturbation of the baseline with continuous deflection of a prolonged activation complex over a 10-s recording period"
2. "with a very short cycle length ($\leq$120 ms) averaged over a 10-s recording period."

Beyond this definition each physician has his/her own interpretation and understanding what a CFAE is and looks like. From clinical practice there is the observation that there are clearly different types of CFAE signals [103].

4.2.1 CFAE Classes in Case of Persistent AF

As observed by physicians, there are varying types of CFAEs that have different importance to the ablation process [103]. From discussions with physicians at Städtisches Klinikum Karlsruhe three types of fractionated signals (C1, C2, C3) that are identified during the ablation procedure are extracted (fig. 4.3). A fourth type (C0) is an also common, but non-fractionated electrogram. These types can be described as

C0: non-fractionated atrial electrogram with high frequency
C1: fractionated atrial electrogram with periodic activity
C2: mixture of periodic fractionated and periodic non-fractionated atrial electrograms
C3: high frequency atrial electrogram with continuous activity

A schematic representation as well as measured signals for each CFAE class is depicted in fig 4.3.
The importance of each class during the ablation process is depending on the history of signals measured at a position while ablating. There is no general rule that, for example, C2 is more important than C3. Nevertheless, usually C3 or C2 signals are more interesting for the ablation process while ablating the fibrillating substrate than signals of class C0.

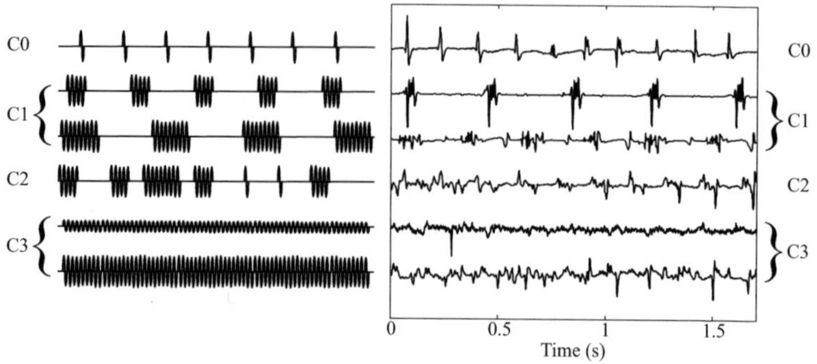

Fig. 4.3: Common CFAEs occurring during an ablation procedure of AF. On the left a schematic representation is depicted and on the right corresponding measured signals. C0 is a non-fractionated atrial electrogram of high frequency, C1 is a fractionated atrial electrogram with periodic activity, C2 is a mixture of periodic fractionated and periodic non-fractionated atrial electrograms, and C3 is a high frequency atrial electrogram with continuous activity.

4.3 Setting up Databases of Atrial Signals

4.3.1 Database of CFAEs

To develop as well as to evaluate algorithms that work on CFAEs, a CFAE database is required. Together with physicians from Städtisches Klinikum Karlsruhe signals during the ablation process of atrial flutter and atrial fibrillation are recorded. Signals from 11 patients who suffered from atrial fibrillation have been recorded semi-automatically. Eight patients suffered from persistent and three patients from paroxysmal AF. All patients were sent to hospital for catheter ablation.
Intracardiac EGM recordings from a multipolar circular catheter such as Lasso (10 polar, Biosense Webster, Diamond Bar, USA), Optima (14 polar, St. Jude Medical, St. Paul, USA), or Orbiter (14 polar, Bard Electrophysiology, Lowell, USA) were performed after pulmonary vein isolation. In addition to the signals the xyz-coordinates of the catheter electrodes and the geometry of the atrium were exported. All together 2824 signals have been exported.
Each recording has a length of 5 seconds and was sampled with 1.2 kHz. The data was prefiltered by the measurement system with a high pass at 30 Hz and a low pass at 250 Hz. Although the data was prefiltered there was sometimes baseline wander or high frequency disturbance left in the signals. Therefore, all measured data was preprocessed with the same filter settings as in the recording system to remove remaining noise (sec. 4.4).

After removing noise by means of signal processing, all signals have been checked visually. Signals that were superimposed with ventricular far field or with ablation artifacts have been sorted out. Signals that were not stationary over 5 seconds were also rejected. Following this process 1417 stationary 5-second signals remained (tab. 4.1).

Table 4.1: Reduction of automatically measured CFAEs by rejecting noisy or non-stationary signals and annotation by two physicians.

	number of signals
all measured signals	2824
signals left for classification	1417
signals rejected by physician	812
classified signals	605
coinciding classification	429

These signals have been classified by two physicians from different centers (tab. 4.1). MD A is an experienced electrophysiologist from Städtisches Klinikum Karlsruhe, MD B an experienced electrophysiologist from Hôpital Cardiologique du Haut-Lévèque, Bordeaux. While classifying, MD A sorted out 812 signals with low quality due to extreme low voltage (suspicion of reduced contact or non-contact). The remaining 605 signals have then been classified according to the above defined classes by MD A and MD B. After the classification process signals that have been assigned to the same class by both physicians have been used to build the CFAE database (tab. 4.2).

Table 4.2: Overview of annotated CFAE signals. MD A is a physician from Karlsruhe, MD B a physician from Bordeaux.

CFAE-Class	MD A	MD B	coinciding
C0	156	154	144
C1	107	143	84
C2	263	191	148
C3	79	117	53

4.3.2 Database of CFAEmean Maps

During the collaboration with the physicians from Städtisches Klinikum Karlsruhe the influence of pulmonary vein isolation (PVI) on the fractionation distribution in the left atrium was investigated. Therefore, CFAEmean maps (sec. 2.4.2) of 27 patients before and after pulmonary vein isolation were recorded with the EnSite NavX™ system. CFAEmean stands for the mean cycle length of local activity. The method how to calculate the value CFAEmean for a given EGM is explained in detail in section 7.5.1. A CFAEmean map consists of the atrial geometry, the measured and evaluated signals and the resulting CFAEmean value for each signal. Maps were regularly recorded during EP study. All together 7849 signals before PVI (290 averaged per patient) and 9654 signals after PVI (357 averaged per patient) were extracted (signal length: 5 seconds).

Table 4.3: Number of datasets of the CFAEmean map database.

	No. of maps	No. of signals
before PVI	27	7849
after PVI	27	9654

For each measurement point only signals that have not been automatically sorted out by the EnSite NavX™ system have been exported. Regularly, these throwouts are signals that have too low or too high amplitude and are recognized as disturbed or noisy signals. The remaining signals have been preprocessed as described in section 4.4.

4.3.3 Database of Contact & Non-Contact Signals

To develop an algorithm that can differentiate between contact and non-contact EGMs another database of EGMs is required. Contact EGMs are signals that have been measured with the catheter having contact to the endocardium and non-contact electrograms that have no or insufficient contact to the endocardium. Signals from 4 patients who suffered from atrial fibrillation (2), atrial flutter, and Wolff-Parkinson-White syndrom have been recorded to build the database. All patients were sent to hospital for catheter ablation.
To reflect different signal morphologies of different regions within the atria, data was acquired in the right atrium (Crista Terminalis, lateral isthmus, medial isthmus, bundle of HIS) and the left atrium (roof, septum, RSPV ostium, anterior

wall). Intracardiac EGM recordings from a 4-pole mapping catheter were performed in sinus rhythm. Bipolar signals from the distal and second electrode have been used. The distance from the distal electrode to the endocardium (pressure, contact, non-contact) was judged by the physician during the measurement through well defined "pull back" maneuvers.
Each recording has a length of around 10 seconds and was sampled with 1 kHz. The data was prefiltered by the measurement system with a high pass at 30 Hz and a low pass at 250 Hz (LABSYSTEM™ PRO EP). All measured data was preprocessed as described in section 4.4. Each signal has been segmented into active segments with the NLEO-based segmenting algorithm (sec. 6.3). The segment length was in the range from 47 ms to 125 ms (mean 82.2 ms). All together 256 segments of contact and non-contact segments (149 contact and 107 non-contact) were exported.

Table 4.4: Number of contact and non-contact EGMs of the contact/non-contact database.

	number of segments
contact	149
non-contact	107

4.4 Preprocessing Atrial Electrograms

All used data was exported from clinical cases. That means data was recorded by commercial systems used in the electrophysiology lab. Systems from which data was exported are

- LABSYSTEM™ PRO EP (C. R. Bard, Inc., Lowell, MA, USA)
- EnSite NavX™ (St. Jude Medical, St. Paul, MN, USA)
- CARTO (Biosense Webster, Diamond Bar, CA, USA)

The data is recorded by these systems with a sample frequency of 1 kHz (LABSYSTEM™ PRO EP) or 1.2 kHz (EnSite NavX™, CARTO) and has been prefiltered. The exported data often remains disturbed with high frequency noise and/or baseline wander. Due to these disturbances the data must be filtered before starting any analysis. Another kind of disturbance is the ventricular far field (VFF), due to the close distance to the ventricles. This VFF can taint the atrial signal depending on the measurement position in the atria. The preprocessing method of denoising atrial signals will be presented in the following section. First, a method to reduce baseline wander is introduced, followed by a high frequency noise reduction algorithm. The ventricular far field removal then is described in chapter 5.

4.4.1 Baseline Wander Removal

Baseline wander is the slow movement of the isoelectric line in an ECG. It can be caused by patient movement, for example chest movement caused by breathing or coughing, poor electrode contact, or interference or drift of the reference potential [7, 104]. Usually, the frequency components of baseline wander are below 2 Hz. Removal of these low frequency parts with a high pass filter is, therefore, possible as no relevant frequency information of the ECG is in this region. In the literature, there are described various algorithms that remove baseline wander from the ECG [105, 106]. In the scope of this work the algorithm developed by Khawaja [104] is used. This algorithm is based on discrete wavelet transform and uses the method of wavelet filter banks (sec. 3.6.1). It has the advantage of reconstructing the biosignal with correlation rates of 99%.
The signal is decomposed with wavelet Daubechie 11 into details and approximations up to level n according to the cut off frequency f_{cut} and the sample frequency f_s. The level is calculated by $n = \mathrm{ld}(f_s/f_{\mathrm{cut}})$. For a cut off frequency of 2 Hz and a sample frequency of 1000 Hz the signal would be decomposed up to level 9. The frequency range that is represented by the level 9 approximation is in the range of 0 and 1.95 Hz. This approximation corresponds to baseline wander in ECG signals [104]. The approximations of this level are set to zero and the signal is composed again by use of IWT.
Figure 4.4 shows an atrial electrogram before and after applying the wavelet transform based baseline wander removal. On the upper figure the signal is tainted with a prominent baseline wander, whereas the baseline wander is removed from the signal on the figure in the middle. The lower figure shows the approximation of the wavelet decomposition of level 10 which corresponds to the baseline wander.

4.4.2 High Frequency Noise Reduction

Signal disturbance in higher frequency ranges is called high frequency noise. The origin of high frequency noise is manifold. Removal of high frequency noise can be achieved by low pass filtering with a cut off frequency at higher levels. In this

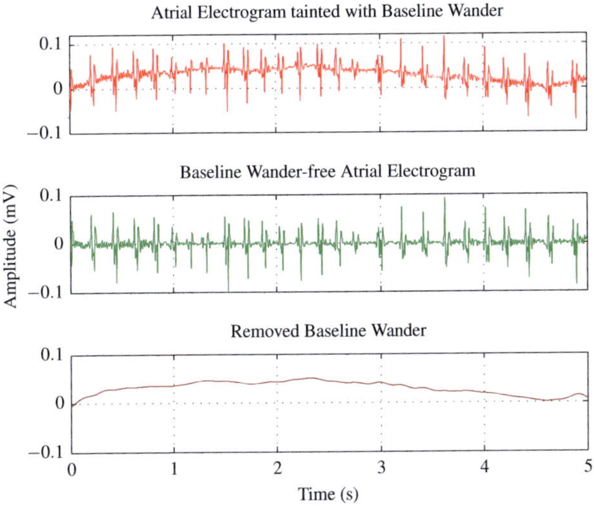

Fig. 4.4: Atrial electrogram tainted with baseline wander (red). After applying the wavelet-based baseline wander removal algorithm [104] with Daubechie's wavelet order 11 up to level 10, the baseline wander (brown) is removed from the signal leading to an iso-electric line (green).

work an adaptive wavelet-based algorithm is used [104]. The denoising implementation of Khawaja is based on the denoising algorithm by Donoho [107]. The advantage of this method is, that rising edges and high energetic peaks in the signal are preserved [79, 104].

It is assumed, that the energy of the noise component is much smaller than the energy of the signal. To denoise the signal it is decomposed with wavelet Daubechie 1 up to the same level as used for the baseline wander removal (sec. 4.4.1). After the decomposition each detail in each level is thresholded by an adaptive threshold [107]. Every part of the details that is beneath the threshold is assumed to represent the noise and is set to zero. The higher energy levels representing the signal's content remain unaffected. Finally, the signal is composed again without the noisy components by use of IWT. Figure 4.5 shows an atrial electrogram tainted with high frequency disturbance before and after applying the high frequency filter.

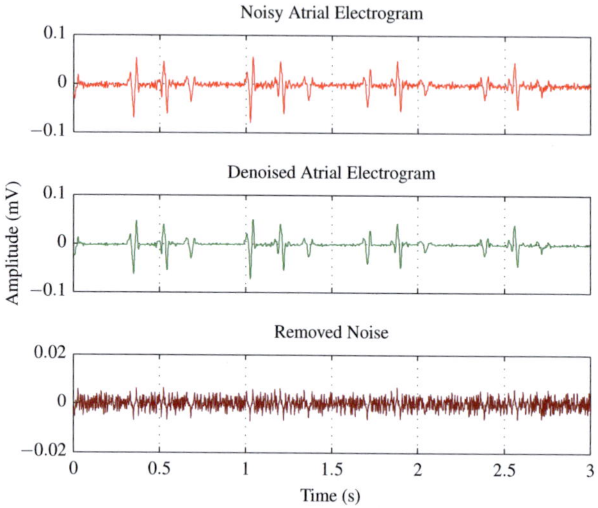

Fig. 4.5: Atrial electrogram tainted with high frequency noise (red). After applying the wavelet-based denoising algorithm [104] with Daubechie's wavelet order 1 up to level 10, the high frequency noise (brown) is removed from the signal leading to a denoised atrial electrogram (green).

5

PCA-based Ventricular Far Field Cancellation

When atrial electrograms are measured in close proximity to the ventricles they can be tainted with ventricular activity [108]. The ventricular activity is superimposed on the atrial activity and is called ventricular far field (VFF). This disturbance of the atrial signals occurs especially in regions of the left atrium like the inferior anterior wall, the inferior posterior wall, or the coronary sinus. The ventricular disturbance pose a problem to signal analysis, especially to rhythmicity analysis (sec. 7.5.3.). An example for ventricular far fields is depicted in figure 5.1. The upper lead shows the surface ECG for comparison. Lead 2 – 5 are bipolar signals measured in the coronary sinus. The ventricular activity is marked with red rectangles. The VFF is most dominant in CS 1/2 and is decreasing in the remaining leads according to increasing distance to the ventricle [3]. As the signal components (atrial and ventricular) origin from different sources it is possible to separate them. Aim of this chapter is to present a method that cancels VFF from a tainted atrial activity.

5.1 The Ventricular Far Field

The VFF is a superposition of the atrial signal. For sinus rhythm the ventricles are triggered by the atrial excitation, more precisely by the sinus node. Therefore, the VFF will follow an atrial activity with regularity. In this case atrial and ventricular activity can be separated easily as they do not occur at the same time. During atrial flutter the atrial frequency is increasing. When the frequency is too fast for the ventricles to follow, the AV node will act as doorman and will allow only each second or third excitation to reach the ventricle [4]. This leads to 2:1 or 3:1 transition. A 3:1 transition is depicted in figure 4.2. In this case, a ventricular activity is only visible after each third atrial activation. If the atria reach more chaotic excita-

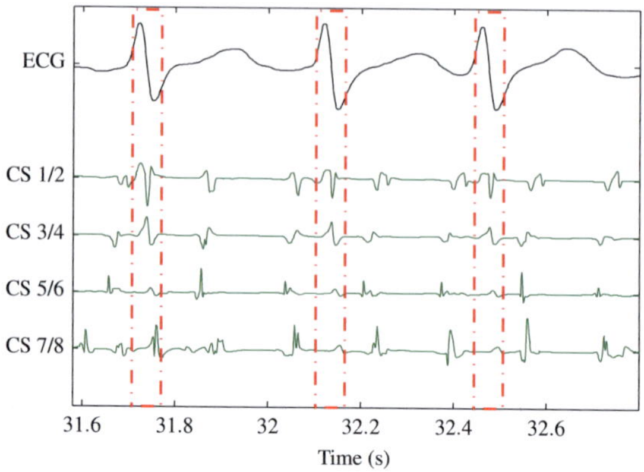

Fig. 5.1: Surface ECG and coronary sinus signals tainted with VFF measured during AF. Ventricular activity is marked with red rectangles.

tions like atrial fibrillation the AV node will take charge of the ventricular rhythm and will act as pacemaker. The atrial excitation and the ventricular excitation are completely decoupled [3,4]. Figure 5.2 shows VFF extracted from 60 seconds of signals measured in the coronary sinus (sec. 11.1). During sinus rhythm (upper left) the amplitude varies only slightly. With increasing atrial frequency the amplitude spread is rising and the regularity is decreasing.

To be able to compare and evaluate the proposed algorithm for cancellation the VFF in atrial EGMs, the energy of the ventricular (E_{VA}) and atrial (E_{AA}) activity will be estimated. Then, based on the concept of signal-to-noise ratio the ventriculo-atrial signal ratio (VASR) is defined as

$$\mathrm{VASR} = 10 \cdot \log_{10}\left(\frac{E_{VA}}{E_{AA}}\right) = 10 \cdot \log_{10}\left(\frac{\sum_i^N s_{VA}^2(i)}{\sum_i^N s_{AA}^2(i)}\right), \tag{5.1}$$

with N the signal length, s_{AA} the pure atrial signal, and s_{VA} the pure ventricular signal. The VASR can differ significantly in dependence of the presence and size of VFF. For signals measured at the coronary sinus the different leads of the CS catheter have been analyzed to reflect the possible range of VASR (tab. 5.1). Lead CS 1/2 usually is closest to the ventricles and has the largest VFF, while CS 7/8 is farthest with small VFF. This is reflected in the mean VASR. CS 1/2 has a mean

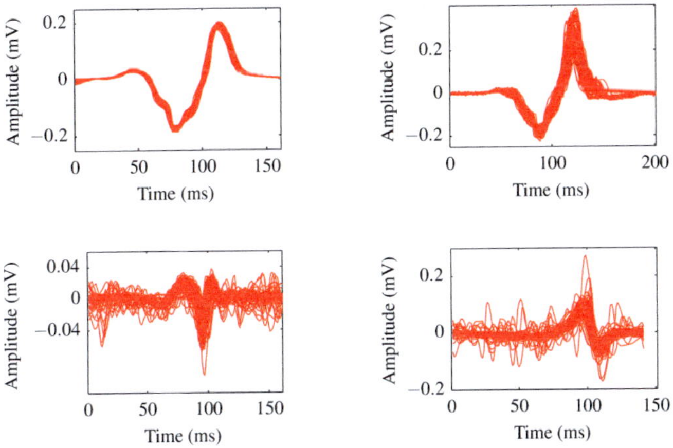

Fig. 5.2: Ventricular far fields during different atrial rhythms. Upper left: Sinus Rhythm, upper right: atrial flutter, lower line: atrial fibrillation case 1 and 2. All signals were measured in the coronary sinus on lead CS 1/2.

VASR of 0.56 dB, whereas the VASR is decreasing from leads CS 3/4 (-7.38 dB) to CS 5/6 (-11.45 dB) and CS 7/8 (-11.48 dB).

Table 5.1: Ventriculo-atrial signal ratio during different atrial rhythms.

Lead	No. of patients	mean VASR (dB)	standard deviation VASR (dB)
CS 1/2	10	0.56	6.74
CS 3/4	10	−7.38	3.87
CS 5/6	10	−11.45	2.48
CS 7/8	10	−11.48	2.71

5.2 Multi-channel PCA-based VFF Reduction

Ventricular far fields do not only occur during EP studies, but also in the surface ECG or in atrial leads of pacemakers. There are different approaches like template matching and subtraction (TMS) [109,110], adaptive ventricular cancellation (AVC) [111], or independent component analysis (ICA) [112] reported in literature to separate ventricular and atrial activity from the ECG or remove ventricular activity from atrial signals.

Rieta and Hornero [111] made a comparative study of the existing ventricular far field cancellation methods. They found that TMS works best for this purpose, but TMS will also deform the atrial signal. ICA by contrast has a better signal fidelity, but performs less well with irregular, disorganized signals. The signals used by Rieta et al. [111, 112] were recorded unipolar at the open epicardial wall after cardiac surgery. They based their algorithms on the assumption that the ventricular far fields tainting the atrial signals have similarity with the QRS complex of the surface ECG. EGMs measured during an EP study are regularly bipolar signals and —especially in case of persistent AF— VFF can vary highly in shape and amplitude according to the measurement position and setup. Additionally, there is no dependency between the shape of QRS complexes of the ECG and VFF. Therefore, the above mentioned methods (ICA and AVC) do not fit the presumptions of atrial signals recorded while EP studies. Although TMS has some shortcomings, it has outperformed the other methods and is used as comparison method.

The method proposed in this chapter is inspired by the work of Castells et al. [113]. In this work ventricular activity has been cancelled out from surface ECG by use of multi-channel independent component analysis. The underlying assumption is that atrial and ventricular activity is uncorrelated while AF and ventricular complexes can be detected in the ECG. Figure 5.3 gives an overview of the fundamental steps of the adapted and improved algorithm to remove VFF from atrial EGMs.

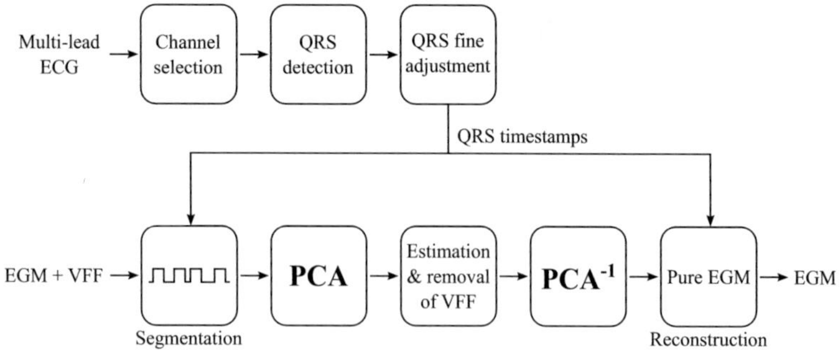

Fig. 5.3: Overview of the algorithm to remove ventricular far field from an EGM.

5.2.1 R-Peak Detection & Segmentation

As the VFF has its origin in the ventricular electrical activity, VFFs occur simultaneously to the QRS complex of the ECG. To remove VFFs from the atrial signal first of all the ventricular activity must be detected. Therefore, the QRS complex is searched in the ECG by use of Pan-Tompkins well established detection algorithm [114]. The number of leads recorded during an EP study is between 3 and 12. The signal's quality within these leads is sometimes varying significantly, due to bad electrode contact, patient movement, or electrical interference. To get the best possible QRS detection results, the mostly undisturbed lead should be chosen for R peak detection.

Undisturbed physiological ECGs consist of P wave, QRS complex, T wave, and to a large extent of iso-electric segments (activity near zero). Computing the amplitude histogram of such an ECG results in a sharp peak around zero and thin tails. Whereas, a broad distribution with large tails in the amplitude histogram is given for noisy ECGs, mainly caused by a disturbed iso-electric line. This behavior is reflected by the excess of the amplitude histogram (sec. 3.1.2 and sec. 3.1.4). The excess will give large values for undisturbed ECGs and smaller or negative values for noisy ECGs [115].

During EP studies even regular, undisturbed ECGs can be tainted with high frequency artifacts at certain times when turning on or off the ablation current. For these cases the excess can be ambiguous. To overcome this ambiguity the excess is calculated on small segments of the ECG and the mean excess for one ECG is determined.

$$\overline{\text{Excess}}(x) = \frac{1}{N}\sum_{i=0}^{N} \text{Excess}(x\,|\,i\cdot T \leq x \leq (i+1)\cdot T) \tag{5.2}$$

N is denoted the number of segments and T the length of each segment. The challenge to choose the best T is, to choose T long enough to include at least one heart cycle and short enough to decrease the influence of artifacts. Here, T is chosen to be one second.

On basis of its excess value the ECG with the largest excess is considered to be the best for QRS detection. With the algorithm introduced by Pan-Tompkins [114] the QRS complexes within the ECG are detected. The ventricular activity inside a time window of $\pm 180\,\text{ms}$ is extracted and a fine adjustment is done to get a better synchronicity between the QRS complexes. The fine adjustment is done within a window of ± 50 ms around the R-peak using Pearson's correlation coefficient. The corrected R-peak position for each QRS complex is then used to detect and extract the ventricular far field inside a time window of ± 180 ms around the corrected R-peak from the EGM.

5.2.2 VFF Removal

In the scope of this method, PCA is used as blind source separation method with positive logic. Blind source separation is a method to extract a set of signals from a mixture of these signals, without knowing how a particular signal contributes to the mixture. The mixture can be modeled as

$$\mathbf{r}(t) = \mathbf{A} \cdot \mathbf{s}(t), \tag{5.3}$$

with the recorded signals denoted $\mathbf{r}(t)$ and the original signals $\mathbf{s}(t)$. The task of blind source separation is to estimate the original signals and the mixing matrix $\mathbf{A}$ based on the recorded signals. Positive logic in this context means, a signal can be either there (coefficient in mixing matrix > 0) or not (coefficient in mixing matrix $= 0$). Because PCA calculation removes the mean value from the signal vector, the mean value is artificially set to zero and transfered into the first principle component. This is done by adding the negative signal vector to the original signal vector. Let $\mathbf{X}$ be the vector of extracted signals of VFF with underlying atrial activity,

$$\mathbf{X} = [x_0, x_1, \ldots, x_N]^T, \tag{5.4}$$

then the input vector for the PCA is $\mathbf{X}^*$

$$\mathbf{X}^* = \begin{bmatrix} \mathbf{X} \\ -\mathbf{X} \end{bmatrix}. \tag{5.5}$$

The mean of $\mathbf{X}^*$ now equals zero and the former mean value is part of the signal variance and will be found in the first principle components. A similar method was used by Sameni et al. to achieve a symmetric point-distribution function prior to independent component analysis in fetal ECG processing [116].
A PCA is applied on the vector $\mathbf{X}^*$ and the obtained eigenvalues (EV) and their related eigenvectors $\mathbf{s}$ are ordered by decreasing component variance. That implies, that the leading EVs represent the highest signal variance. Since the VFF are similar in shape in all extracted segments and for each atrial rhythm (fig. 5.2), they

will be represented by the leading EVs. Atrial signals can be considered as singular, especially for persistent atrial fibrillation. Thus, the VFF representation in the principal component scores matrix ψ is decreasing with decrementing eigenvalues. On the other hand, the most significant atrial signals are combined into the least significant ventricular signals.

$$\mathbf{X}^* = \psi \cdot \mathbf{s}^\mathbf{T} = \begin{bmatrix} \psi_{\text{ventricle},0} \\ \psi_{\text{ventricle},1} \\ \vdots \\ \psi_{\text{ventricle},n-i} + \psi_{\text{atrium},0} \\ \psi_{\text{ventricle},n-(i-1)} + \psi_{\text{atrium},1} \\ \vdots \\ \psi_{\text{ventricle},n} + \psi_{\text{atrium},i} \\ \psi_{\text{atrium},i+1} \\ \vdots \\ \psi_{\text{atrium},m} \end{bmatrix} \cdot \mathbf{s}^\mathbf{T} \tag{5.6}$$

Hence, it is feasible to delete the first EVs with their according eigenvectors to remove the ventricular far field. The remaining signal parts are then the ones that belong to atrial activity.

$$\mathbf{X}^*_{\text{filtered}} = \psi \cdot \begin{bmatrix} 0 & & & & \\ & \ddots & & & \\ & & 0 & & \\ & & & 1 & & \\ & & & & \ddots & \\ & & & & & 1 \end{bmatrix} \cdot \mathbf{s}^\mathbf{T} \tag{5.7}$$

The challenge is now to remove enough eigenvalues to suppress the ventricular activity without deleting atrial signal parts. Table 5.2 shows the explained variance for the first three eigenvalues for different atrial rhythms. Assume that it is sufficient to remove more than 90% of explained variance. In case of SR and AFlut it is sufficient to remove only the first eigenvalue as the explained variance is 98.8% and 92.9%, respectively. In case of AF_I the first five EVs are needed to give a cumulative sum of explained variances around 90%. Even nine EVs are needed in case of AF_2. Setting a hard threshold will not lead to satisfying results as the spread of needed EVs is too big.

Table 5.2: Explained variance of first three eigenvalues for different atrial rhythms.

	Lead	No.	$\lambda_1/\sum_i \lambda_i$	$\lambda_2/\sum_i \lambda_i$	$\lambda_3/\sum_i \lambda_i$
SR	CS1 unipolar	56	98.9%	0.7%	0.1%
AFlut	CS2 unipolar	109	92.9%	3.5%	1.6%
AF_1	CS 1/2	114	76.4%	9.0%	1.8%
AF_2	CS 1/2	97	57.3%	8.7%	5.3%

The VASR reflects the ratio of ventricular activity to atrial activity. For unknown signals the VASR is estimated. Therefore, the “pure” ventricular signal is estimated by applying a PCA on the extracted ventricular activity as described above. The first two principle components are assumed to represent the VFF. The “pure” atrial signal is estimated from the activity not falling into the R-peak marked windows. Based on these signals the VASR is estimated. Large values imply large VFF, whereas small values imply small or non atrial activity. For large VFF (large VASR) the ventricular activity will be represented by a number of principle components. The less atrial activity is existing, the more principle components will represent VFF. Thus, the number of components to be deleted can be associated with the VASR. For small VASR values only the first component will reflect ventricular activity. With increasing VASR also the number of components to delete must be increased. During simulations a step function of number of principle components to delete was found to give good results. Table 5.3 shows the values chosen for the step function.

Table 5.3: Number of PCA components to delete based on VASR.

Range	No. of components
$\mathrm{VASR} < -5\,\mathrm{dB}$	1
$-5\,\mathrm{dB} \leq \mathrm{VASR} < 0\,\mathrm{dB}$	2
$0\,\mathrm{dB} \leq \mathrm{VASR} < 5\,\mathrm{dB}$	3
$\mathrm{VASR} \geq 5\,\mathrm{dB}$	5

Another criterion, to chose the number of principles components to delete, can be the excess. The basic assumption to use this criterion is, that atrial and ventricular activity are uncorrelated. As the segments are synchronized to the QRS complex, each segment should contain ventricular activity. The PCA scores belonging to the first eigenvalue, therefore, should contain the representation of ventricular activity. Calculating a histogram on these scores leads to a more uniform distribution than scores representing atrial activity. The latter build a more spiky histogram. This behavior can be described by the excess (sec. 3.1.4). Thus, small excess values belong to VFF and high excess values to atrial activity and the excess can be used to distinguish between VFF and atrial activity. While evaluating the success of excess based selection of components to delete, it turned out, that it has a generally good performance, but sometimes outliers occur and can even lead to a significant impairment, since sometimes the number of components selected was too large. Finally, a combination of VASR and excess criterions was implemented. The VASR criterion is used to set the upper limit to the number of components selected for deletion, while the excess criterion sets the actual number, if the limit is not reached.

After removing the components belonging to the ventricular far field, the PCA scores are transformed back into time domain and the signal parts which have been cut out at the beginning are replaced with the remaining atrial signal parts.

5.3 Evaluation Method

The best way to evaluate the proposed method would be to measure the pure atrial signal, the pure VFF, and the superimposed signal and to compare the cancellation results with the pure original signals. Unfortunately, it is not possible to record atrial activity separated from VFF in the atria. So, the golden truth is unknown. Using pure synthetic signals to evaluate the method may not give reliable signals, as they do not necessarily reflect the golden truth. But, artificial signals can be used to estimate the validity of the proposed VFF cancellation method. Because of this, real VFF are artificially superimposed to pure atrial activity to achieve test signals.

Pure atrial activity was gained from lead CS 7/8 from a catheter placed in the coronary sinus. The physicians took care to record a signal that was not tainted with VFF. Ventricular activity while AF can vary greatly in shape (fig. 5.2). To reflect this variety, not only one VFF is taken into account. A set of ventricular activity is used to generate different VFF. These different ventricular far fields have been extracted during sinus rhythm and atrial flutter from CS 1/2 with the method in-

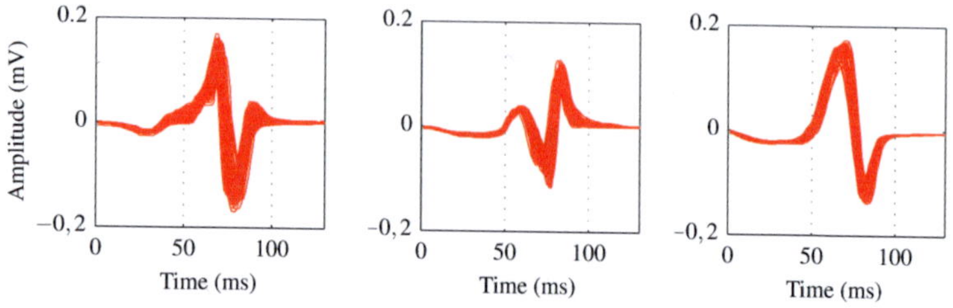

Fig. 5.4: Measured VFF to evaluate the ventricular far field cancellation method. The left and the middle signal have been measured during atrial flutter and the right signal during sinus rhythm.

troduced in section 11.1 (fig. 5.4). Additionally, a synthetic ventricular signal is generated for which amplitude and signal variance is known. The synthetic VFF is used to have a signal with known variance and to have a signal that can be adjusted to test the sufficient deletion of PCA components. The synthetic signal simulates a VFF found in recordings on lead CS 1/2. It is built from a base shape and second order variance (fig. 5.5). The base shape s_{base} is obtained by

$$s_{\text{base}}(n) = \begin{cases} 0 & \text{for } n \leq 20 \\ (n-20)\cdot\sin\left[55\cdot\pi/28\cdot(n-20)^2\right] & \text{for } 21 \leq n \leq 70 \\ 50\cdot\sin\left[55\cdot\pi/28\cdot(n-20)^2\right] & \text{for } 71 \leq n \leq 90 \\ -25\cdot\exp[-(n-91)/80] & \text{for } 91 \leq n \leq 171 \end{cases} \tag{5.8}$$

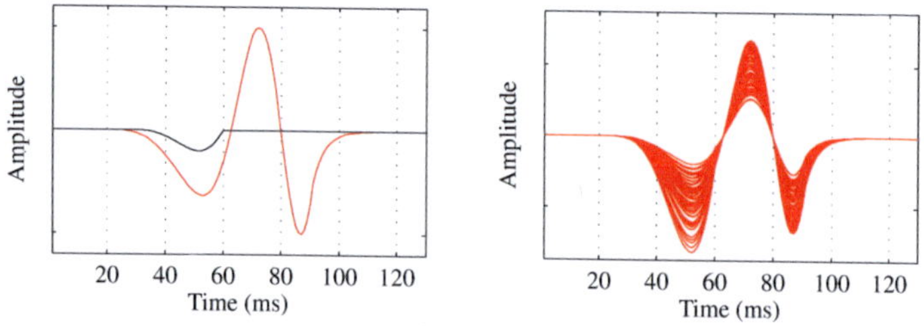

Fig. 5.5: Synthetic VFF to evaluate the ventricular far field cancellation method. On the left hand side the base shape (red) and the second order variance are depicted. On the right hand side a variation of constructed VFF is shown.

The second order variance s_{var} is implemented by:

$$s_{var}(n) = \begin{cases} 0 & \text{for } n \leq 30 \\ -10 \cdot \sin\left(\pi/30 \cdot (n-31)^2\right) & \text{for } 31 \leq n \leq 60 \\ 0 & \text{for } 61 \leq n \leq 171 \end{cases} \tag{5.9}$$

For the evaluation of the algorithm at least one surface ECG is needed to detect the ventricular activity. Therefore, mean QRS complexes in two leads (II, V1) are calculated. An artificial ventricular heart rate with a mean frequency of 85 beats per minute was generated. An arrhythmia of ± 200 ms was included to give a more realistic ECG while AF. This heart rate and the extracted mean QRS complexes were used to generate two leads of surface ECG (II and V1). An example of one used QRS complex can be seen in figure 5.6.

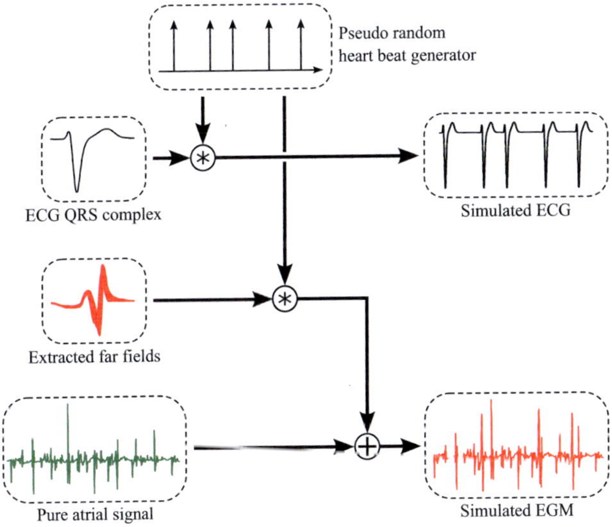

Fig. 5.6: Generating test signals for the evaluation of VFF removal algorithm.

With the presented signals, test signals for the evaluation have been generated. Figure 5.6 gives an overview of building the evaluation signals. The artificial heart rate specifies the occurrence of ventricular activity. The pure atrial signal was superimposed with ventricular activity according to the heart rate. Thus, an ECG and a VFF tainted atrial electrogram were obtained.

The evaluation of the proposed method is based on how closely the algorithm will reconstruct the atrial signal before superimposition. Therefore, the pure atrial signal will be correlated with the reconstructed atrial activity. As a measure for the similarity of the signals the cross correlation coefficient ρ (eq. (3.11)) was used.

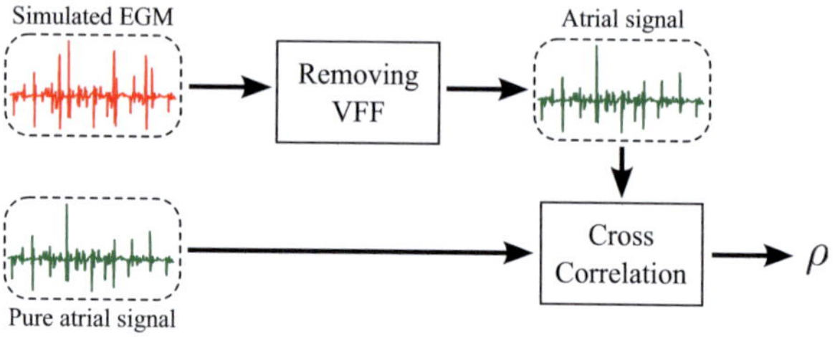

Fig. 5.7: Evaluation of VFF removal algorithm.

5.4 Results of Ventricular Far Field Cancellation

Before discussing the results of the evaluation method, first a proof of concept on a real measured signal is shown. Figure 5.8 depicts an VFF tainted signal (red curve) and the same signal after removing VFF (green curve). Ventricular activity is marked by detecting the QRS complex (blue dots). It can be seen, that instead of the removed VFF, atrial activity is visible. This is the recovered atrial activity, which was originally superimposed by the VFF.

To evaluate the outcome of the proposed approach to remove VFFs, this approach is compared to the TMS method (blue curves) and the result, when no filter is applied (black curve). For the latter the pure atrial signal is cross correlated with the unchanged superimposed signal. The correlation coefficient ρ is calculated for different values of VASR, to reflect the methods outcome for different sized VFF. The methods are applied on the different artificial signals described in the preceding section and results are shown for different criteria to decide how many principle components will be removed. Additionally, to the introduced VASR criterion, the excess criterion, and the combination of both criteria, a fixed 2-component reduction was done.

Independent from the test signal, the fixed 2-component criterion shows inferior results for VASR values below -5 dB compared to the TMS method (fig. 5.9 (a),

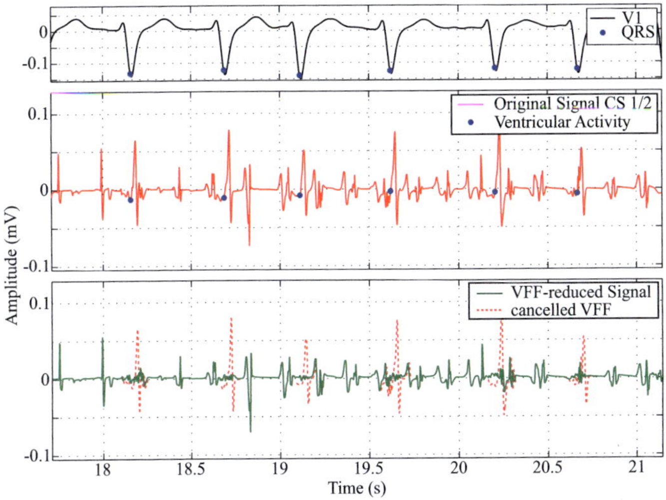

Fig. 5.8: Surface ECG (V1, black), original coronary sinus signal (red) and the sole atrial coronary sinus signal (green) with superimposed cancelled ventricular far field (dotted, red).

5.10 (a), 5.11 (a), and 5.12 (a)). Instead for large VASR the 2-component criterion is superior to the TMS. For signals containing only a small number of VFF components, like during sinus rhythm (fig. 5.12 (a)), it is good choice to remove two components, and thus, the results are steady for the complete range of VASR.

Comparing the excess criterion with the TMS method (fig. 5.9 (c), 5.10 (c), 5.11 (c), and 5.12 (c)), one can state, that the excess criterion is inferior in the range beneath −5 dB, but as the mean difference is smaller than 0.02, this difference is negligible. For VASR larger than −5 dB the excess criterion performs better than the TMS method. Excepting the AFlut signal case 2, the excess criterion performs better or equal compared to the VASR criterion. The VASR criterion gives generally good results, even for signals that have rather small variance. Compared to the TMS method the VASR criterion gives similar results for VASR values smaller than −5 dB. With increasing VASR the VASR criterion is superior (fig. 5.9 (c), 5.10 (c), 5.11 (c)). In figures 5.9 (c), 5.11 (c), and 5.12 (c), the applied step function of the VASR criterion is visible. Steps around 0 dB and 5 dB can be observed. For, e.g. the synthetic signal (fig. 5.9 (c)), the ventricular signal does not contain a large number of variances. Thus, each step of the VASR criterion's step function

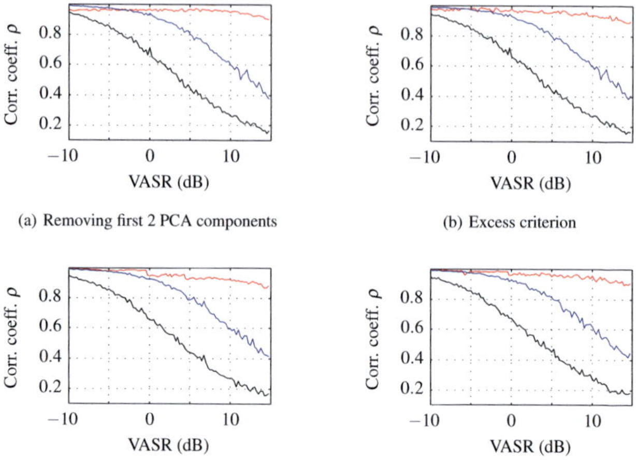

(a) Removing first 2 PCA components

(b) Excess criterion

(c) VASR criterion

(d) Excess + VASR

Fig. 5.9: Evaluation of synthetic VFF cancellation. The result of PCA-based VFF reduction is depicted in red, the result of the TMS method in blue, and the result of the unmodified signal in black.

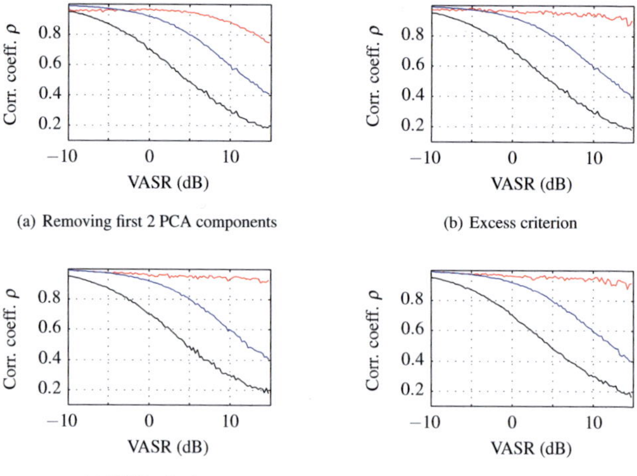

(a) Removing first 2 PCA components

(b) Excess criterion

(c) VASR criterion

(d) Excess + VASR

Fig. 5.10: Evaluation of AFlut case 1 VFF cancellation. The result of PCA-based VFF reduction is depicted in red, the result of the TMS method in blue, and the result of the unmodified signal in black.

(tab. 5.3) leads to a decrease in the correlation coefficient, because, atrial signal parts have been removed, too. VASR might by a good criterion to limit the amount of components to delete, if the excess criterion fails and selects a too large number. The interaction of both criteria can be seen in figure 5.11 and figure 5.12. For the AFlut case 2 signal (fig. 5.11) the excess criterion gives poor results for large VASR. This result can be improved by combining excess and VASR criterion (fig. 5.11 (d)). Indeed in this example sole VASR would give the best result. However, examining the sinus rhythm signal (fig. 5.12) leads to best results for the excess criterion and the combined criterion. Comparing the results for all given test signals, the combination of VASR criterion and excess criterion results in the best outcome for the whole range of VASR.

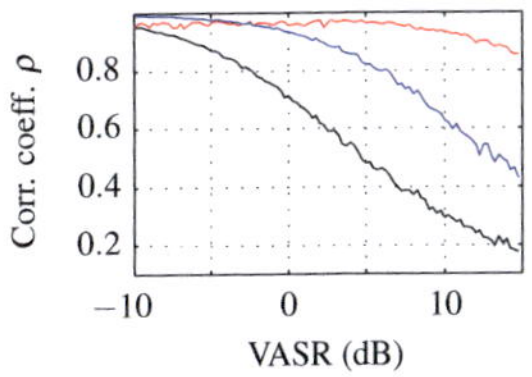

(a) Removing first 2 PCA components

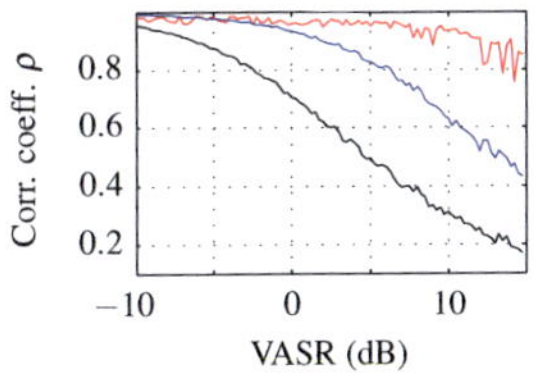

(b) Excess criterion

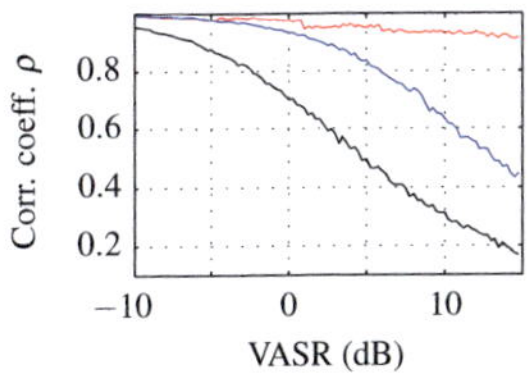

(c) VASR criterion

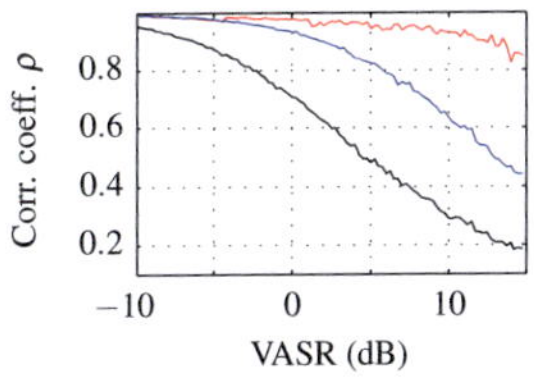

(d) Excess + VASR

Fig. 5.11: Evaluation of AFlut case 2 VFF cancellation. The result of PCA-based VFF reduction is depicted in red, the result of the TMS method in blue, and the result of the unmodified signal in black.

Concluding, the combination of VASR criterion and the excess criterion performs better than the TMS-method for all values of VASR. Thus, the new proposed PCA-based method to remove ventricular far fields works better than the TMS method. As there are no other methods to remove the VFF from atrial signals described in literature, this method improves the possibility to preprocess superimposed atrial electrograms. Thus, subsequently used descriptors will perform better, as the results are not ambiguous because of interpreting the VFF as well. This will lead to

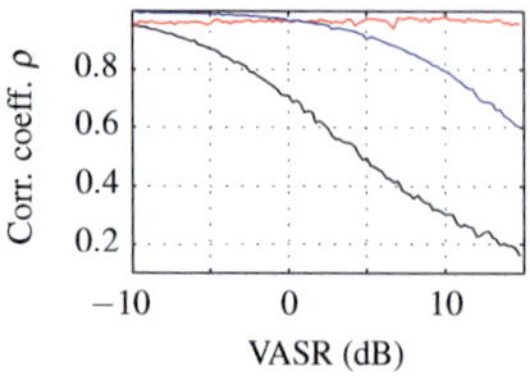

(a) Removing first 2 PCA components

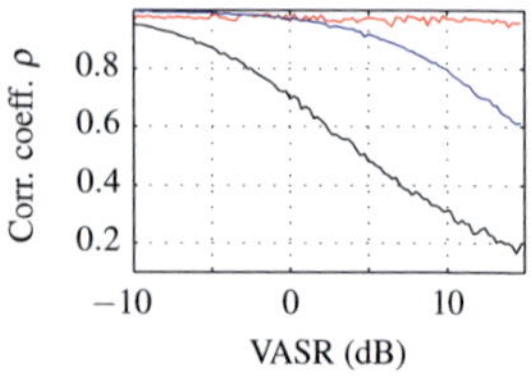

(b) Excess criterion

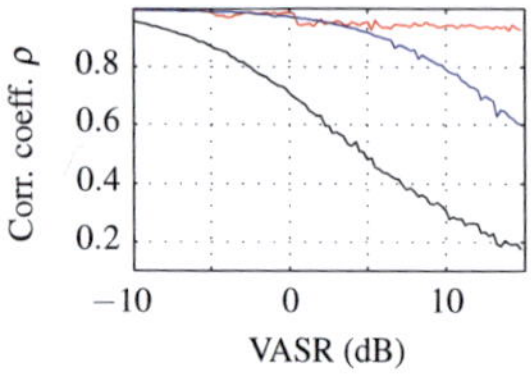

(c) VASR criterion

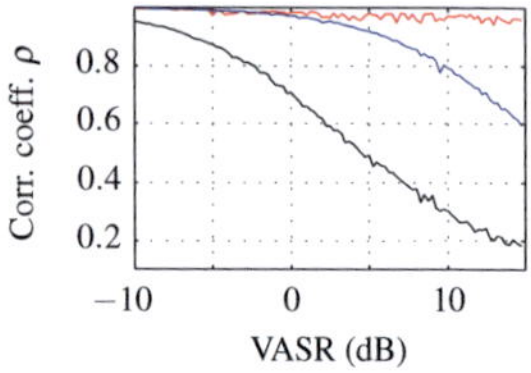

(d) Excess + VASR

Fig. 5.12: Evaluation of SR VFF cancellation. The result of PCA-based VFF reduction is depicted in red, the result of the TMS method in blue, and the result of the unmodified signal in black.

more reliable outcomes, when analyzing and investigating CFAEs and the atrial substrate.

6

Segmenting Atrial Electrograms

Interpreting atrial electrograms during catheter ablation is an important process to achieve sustainable ablation success. Therefore, EGMs are interpreted visually by the physician. One main task is to decide between active and inactive segments within a signal stream. This is a tricky exercise as, especially in atrial fibrillation, there is no isoelectric line. Here, the main task is to separate the signals from noise. The signal analyzing process is addicted distinctly to the physician's experience in the catheter lab. In the following chapter a method is presented that, based on a non-linear energy operator, will separate active and inactive segments in an atrial electrogram.

6.1 Energy of a Harmonic Oscillation

Based on an ideal spring-mass-system with the mass m and the spring constant k, Hooke's law is defined as $F = -kx$. Hooke's law states that the force F with which a spring pushes back is linearly proportional to the distance x from its equilibrium length. According to Newton's law the force F is equal to mass m times acceleration a. The force equation for a spring obeying Hooke's law results in

$$ma = -kx. \tag{6.1}$$

With $a = \ddot{x}$ equation (6.1) leads to a second order linear differential equation for the displacement x as a function of time

$$\ddot{x} + \frac{k}{m}x = 0. \tag{6.2}$$

The solution of this second order differential is given by a harmonic oscillation

$$x(t) = A\cos(\omega t + \phi),$$

where A is the amplitude, $\omega = \sqrt{k/m}$ the angular frequency, and ϕ the phase of the oscillation.

The energy of a mass-spring-system is given by the sum of the kinetic and the potential energy

$$E = \frac{1}{2}kx^2 + \frac{1}{2}m\dot{x}^2. \tag{6.3}$$

Inserting $x(t)$ results in

$$E = \frac{1}{2}m\omega^2 A^2. \tag{6.4}$$

From equation (6.4) follows, that

$$E \propto A^2\omega^2. \tag{6.5}$$

According to equation (6.5) it is obvious that the energy of a mass-spring-system is proportional to the square of the amplitude and the square of the angular frequency.

6.2 Non-Linear Energy Operator

In most cases of signal processing the energy of a signal is calculated as the time integral over the square of the signal's amplitude. For discrete signals the integral changes into a sum [80]. The energy of a time-discrete signal x_n is

$$E_x = \sum_{n=0}^{N} |x_n|^2. \tag{6.6}$$

This definition of the energy of a signal does not regard the frequency content of this signal. Kaiser et al. [117] introduced the non-linear energy operator (NLEO) as an on-the-fly energy calculation of time discrete signals that regards the amplitude as well as the frequency of a given signal. The derivation of the NLEO will be introduced. The complete derivation can be found in [117]. Given is a harmonic oscillation $x(t)$ and its time-discrete representation x_n

$$x_n = A\cos(\Omega n + \phi), \tag{6.7}$$

where A is the amplitude, $\Omega = 2\pi f/f_s$ the digital angular frequency, f the frequency of $x(t)$, f_s the sample frequency, and ϕ the phase of the signal. Equation (6.7) comprises three unknown parameters A, Ω and ϕ. With three sample values of x_n these three unknowns can be calculated. For convenience three adjacent equally-spaced samples were chosen:

$$x_n = A\cos(n\Omega + \phi) \tag{6.8}$$

$$x_{n+1} = A\cos((n+1)\Omega + \phi) \tag{6.9}$$

$$x_{n-1} = A\cos((n-1)\Omega + \phi). \tag{6.10}$$

Using the trigonometric identity [118]

$$\cos(\alpha+\beta)\cos(\alpha-\beta) = \frac{1}{2}(\cos(2\alpha)+\cos(2\beta)), \tag{6.11}$$

the following equation can be obtained for the product $x_{n+1} \cdot x_{n-1}$

$$x_{n+1} \cdot x_{n-1} = \frac{A^2}{2}(\cos(2\Omega n + 2\phi) + \cos(2\Omega)). \tag{6.12}$$

Using more trigonometric identities and doing some substitution, and reformatting of equation (6.12) results in

$$x_n^2 - x_{n+1} \cdot x_{n-1} = A^2 \sin^2 \Omega. \tag{6.13}$$

Equation (6.13) is exact and unique under the restriction that Ω is in the range $(-\pi/2, \pi/2)$. This implies that the maximal frequency f of the signal is less then one-fourth of the sample frequency f_s. For small values of Ω, $\sin(\Omega) \approx \Omega$ holds true

$$x_n^2 - x_{n+1} \cdot x_{n-1} \approx A^2\Omega^2 \tag{6.14}$$

If the values of Ω are limited to $\Omega < \pi/4$, i.e. $f/f_s < 1/8$, then the relative error is smaller than 11% [117]. So the non-linear energy operator is defined as

$$E_{\text{NLEO}} = x_n^2 - x_{n+1} \cdot x_{n-1} \approx A^2\Omega^2. \tag{6.15}$$

Compared with equation (6.5) one can see that the NLEO is an approximation of the energy of an oscillating signal at time n. The NLEO is proportional to the squared amplitude as well as the squared frequency of the signal. Thus, the NLEO is a very fast algorithm to determine a measure of the signal's energy.

To validate the output of the NLEO, the NLEO is tested on common signals with different amplitude and frequency content in the next section. First, the influence of amplitude variations on the NLEO with a damped sinus signal is analyzed. Next, the NLEO is tested with a chirp signal. After that, NLEO's output on two superimposed sinus signals with different frequencies is shown.

6.2.1 NLEO of an Exponentially Damped Sinus Signal

A sinus signal with frequency Ω and amplitude Φ is damped exponentially with e^{-an}:

$$x_n = A\mathrm{e}^{-an}\sin(\Omega n + \Phi). \tag{6.16}$$

That means the amplitude is decreasing exponentially with time while the frequency remains constant. The approximation of the NLEO (6.13) for this signal then is:

$$\begin{aligned} E_{\text{NLEO,damped sinus}} &= A^2 \sin^2 \Omega \\ &= \left(A\mathrm{e}^{-an}\right)^2 \sin^2(\Omega). \end{aligned} \tag{6.17}$$

Assuming that the signal's frequency is less than an eighth of the sample frequency ($\Omega < \pi/4$), the following approximation holds true:

$$E_{\text{NLEO, damped sinus}} \approx \left(A\mathrm{e}^{-an}\right)^2 \Omega^2 = A^2\mathrm{e}^{-2an}\Omega^2. \tag{6.18}$$

The NLEO of a damped sinus with constant frequency Ω decreases with a squared exponential function e^{-2an} (fig. 6.1). With decreasing amplitude, also the NLEO output vanishes.

6.2.2 NLEO of a Chirp Signal

A chirp signal is a signal with constant amplitude but varying frequency. A time discrete chirp signal with a circular frequency starting at $\Omega = \Omega_1$ and increasing linearly by $\Delta\Omega$ after N sample values is defined. Thus, the current frequency of the chirp signal is:

$$\Omega(n) = \Omega_1 \frac{\Delta\Omega}{N} n, \quad n = 1, \ldots, N. \tag{6.19}$$

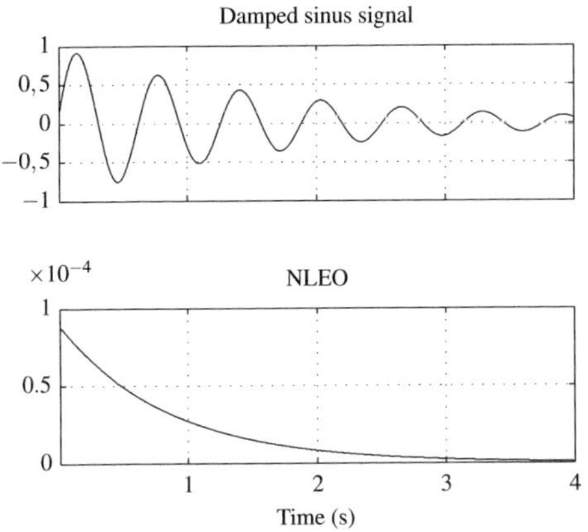

Fig. 6.1: Damped sinus signal with decreasing amplitude and its NLEO. With decreasing amplitude the energy (NLEO) of the damped sinus is also decreasing.

The current phase $\theta(n)$ of the function $A\cos(\Omega(n)\cdot n) = A\cos(\theta(n))$ is given from the integration of the circular frequency $\Omega(k)$

$$\begin{aligned}\theta(n) &= \int_1^n \Omega(k)\mathrm{d}k \\ &= \Omega_1 n - \frac{\Delta\Omega}{2N}n^2. \end{aligned} \tag{6.20}$$

Hence, the chirp signal with a linear frequency shift is

$$x_n = A\cos\left(\Omega_n - \frac{\Delta\Omega}{2N}n^2\right). \tag{6.21}$$

The NLEO of the chirp signal is derived by inserting (6.21) into (6.15).

$$\begin{aligned}E_{\text{NLEO, chirp}} &= x_n^2 - x_{n+1}x_{n-1} \\ &= A^2\cos^2\left(\Omega_1 n - \frac{\Delta\Omega}{2N}n^2\right) \\ &\quad - A^2\cos\left(\Omega_1(n+1) - \frac{\Delta\Omega}{2N}(n+1)^2\right) \\ &\quad \cdot\cos\left(\Omega_1(n-1) - \frac{\Delta\Omega}{2N}(n-1)^2\right)\end{aligned}$$

Using equation (6.20) and (6.21) follows:

$$E_{\text{NLEO, chirp}} = A^2 \cos^2(\theta(n)) \\ - A^2 \cos\left(\theta(n) - \frac{\Delta\Omega}{2N} + \Omega(n)\right) \cos\left(\theta(n) - \frac{\Delta\Omega}{2N} - \Omega(n)\right).$$

Applying some trigonometric identities and assuming a small changing rate of the frequency Ω, the following approximations

$$\frac{\Delta\Omega}{N} \ll 1, \qquad \sin\left(\frac{\Delta\Omega}{2N}\right) \approx \frac{\Delta\Omega}{2N} \qquad \text{and} \qquad \cos\left(\frac{\Delta\Omega}{2N}\right) \approx 1$$

lead to

$$A^2 \sin^2\left(\theta(n) - \frac{\Delta\Omega}{2N}\right) = A^2\left(\sin^2(\theta(n)) - \sin(2\,\theta(n))\frac{\Delta\Omega}{2N}\right).$$

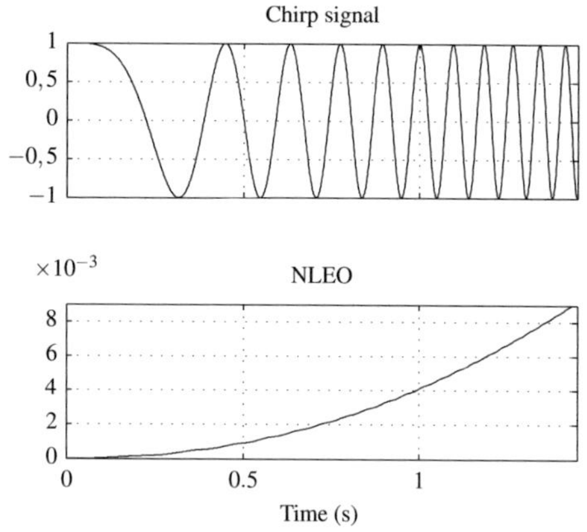

Fig. 6.2: Chirp signal with increasing frequency and its NLEO. With increasing frequency the energy (NLEO) of the chirp signal is rising.

Finally, with $\cos^2\alpha + \sin^2\alpha = 1$ the energy of the chirp signal is:

$$\begin{aligned}
E_{\text{NLEO, chirp}} &= A^2\cos^2(\theta(n)) - A^2 + A^2\left(\sin^2(\theta(n)) - \sin(2\,\theta(n))\frac{\Delta\Omega}{2N}\right) \\
&\quad + A^2\sin^2(\Omega(n)) \\
&= -A^2\sin(2\,\theta(n))\frac{\Delta\Omega}{2N} + A^2\sin^2(\Omega(n)) \\
&\approx A^2\sin^2(\Omega(n)).
\end{aligned}$$

Assuming that the signal's frequency is less than an eighth of the sample frequency ($\Omega < \pi/4$), the energy of the chirp signal can be approximated with:

$$E_{\text{NLEO, chirp}} = A^2\Omega^2(n). \tag{6.22}$$

The chirp signal defined in (6.21) and the NLEO of this signal is depicted in figure 6.2. With increasing frequency also the output of the NLEO is rising.

6.2.3 NLEO of Superimposed Sinus Functions

The last example is a signal of two superimposed sinus signals. Therefore, a sinus with 12 Hz is added to a sinus with 16 Hz. The resulting signal, its envelope, and the NLEO output is shown in fig. 6.3. The NLEO mirrors the trend of the signal's envelope.

6.3 NLEO-based Segmentation of CFAEs

While interpreting and analyzing intracardiac electrograms during an electrophysiological examination, the physician divides the electrogram into active and inactive segments. An active segment is a part of the electrogram where atrial activity is present, whereas an inactive segment is the part of an electrogram where the tissue beneath the electrode is inactive and an iso-electric line or noise is present. Active segments are recognized by high frequency content and large, deflecting amplitudes. This is similar to the surface ECG where the QRS-complex reflects the electrically active part of the heart and the iso-electric line the period of rest. Figure 6.9 depicts examples of signals with different atrial rhythm. The upper case is a sinus rhythm signal, whereas the middle and the lower ones are flutter and fibrillation signals. The differentiation between active and inactive segments

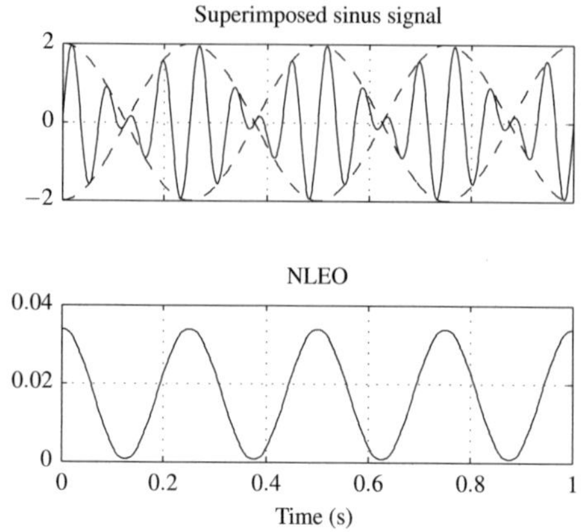

Fig. 6.3: Superimposed sinus signals with 12 Hz and 16 Hz and the NLEO output of the signal. The energy (NLEO) follows the envelope (dashed line) of the superimposed signals.

is obvious for SR and AFlut, but more difficult for the AF case. The separation in active and inactive segments is done by the physician and is based on his/her experience. Based on this separation, the pathological status of the atria is rated and the following ablation procedure is planed.

As the separation of electrograms in active and inactive segments is the bases of following analysis, in this section an algorithm will be introduced to segment electrograms automatically in active and inactive segments. The algorithm is based on Pan-Tompkin's QRS-detection algorithm [114] applied to the output of the NLEO. Instead of using the signals' frequency to separate segments with different activity the change of the signal's energy is used. After removing baseline wander and high frequency disturbance (sec. 4.4) from the electrogram, the energy of the electrogram is computed by use of the NLEO algorithm (sec. 6.2). The NLEO output emphasizes sections with high frequencies and large amplitudes (fig. 6.4).

The pure output of the NLEO is low-pass filtered to smooth the graph. Instead of a sliding window as proposed by Pan-Tompkins, a gaussian low-pass is chosen. The advantage of a gaussian low-pass against a rectangular window is, that both, the amplitude and frequency response, are a gaussian too, and therefore, are smooth in the pass band. According to Pan-Tompkins, the effective width of the impulse response should be chosen in the dimension of the mean width of deflections. The deflections of EGMs are typically in the range of 10 – 20 ms. For a mean width of

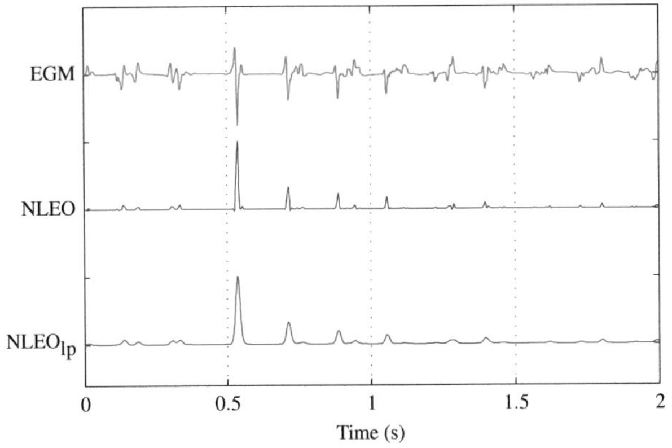

Fig. 6.4: NLEO output of the given EGM. The middle lead depicts the pure NLEO output and the lower lead the low-pass filtered NLEO.

14 ms the effective width of the impulse response will be 17 sample values (sample frequency 1200 Hz). As the interesting frequency range for electrograms is in the range of 0 – 20 Hz [119], the cut-off frequency is set to 24 Hz (fig. 6.5). The output of the gaussian low-pass filter is depicted in figure 6.4 (lower lead).

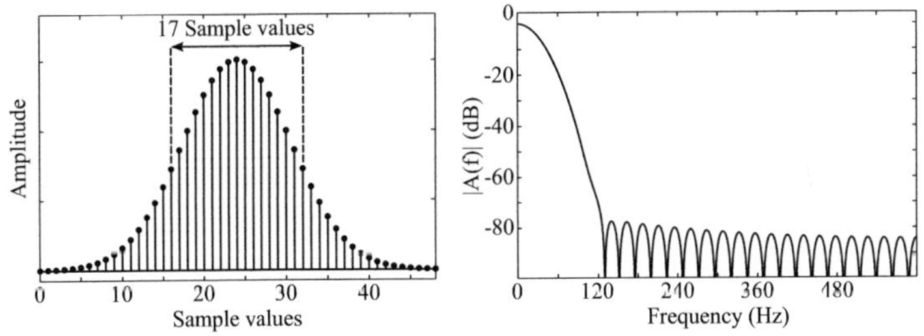

Fig. 6.5: Impulse and frequency response of the gaussian low-pass filter.

Non-zero parts in the low-pass filtered NLEO represent atrial activity. To detect these parts an adaptive thresholding is implemented. The standard deviation of the NLEO as threshold for the detection leads to reasonable results. This threshold will overemphasize large peaks and ignore small peaks. Hence, a windowing is applied to accommodate the dynamics of the NLEOs output (fig. 6.4). The atrial frequency during AF is between 4 – 10 Hz. Applying a window of 1 second will contain 4 – 10 atrial excitations. This is enough data to do statistical analysis, e.g. calculating the standard deviation. The window is moved with $\Delta t = 50\,\text{ms}$. For each data point $x(n)$ 20 thresholds $Y_i(n)$ will be obtained, except the data points within the first and last second. For each data point the minimal threshold is chosen as final threshold $Y_{\text{thresh}}(n)$

$$Y_{\text{thresh}}(n) = \min(Y_i(n)) \qquad i = 1, \ldots, 20. \tag{6.23}$$

In discussions with physicians it turned out, that the best segmentation was achieved when the standard deviation was weighted with a factor $k = 0.1$. Each data point of the NLEO that exceeds its threshold is marked as active, otherwise as inactive. Adjacent points with the same mark are merged. This leads to active and inactive segments. As the NLEO and the original electrogram have the same x-axes, the found segmentation can be applied on the electrogram.
Finally, the electrophysiological validity of the segmentation needs to be proven. A refractory period of 42 ms is defined. This is a reasonable value as it is also regularly used in commercial systems in the EP lab. The gap between two active segments should be larger than 42 ms. Inactive segments that are shorter than this refractory period are ignored and the adjacent active segments are merged. On the other hand marked active segments that are shorter than 10 ms have no physiological meaning and are considered to be inactive. The block diagram of the NLEO-based segmentation algorithm is shown in figure 6.6.

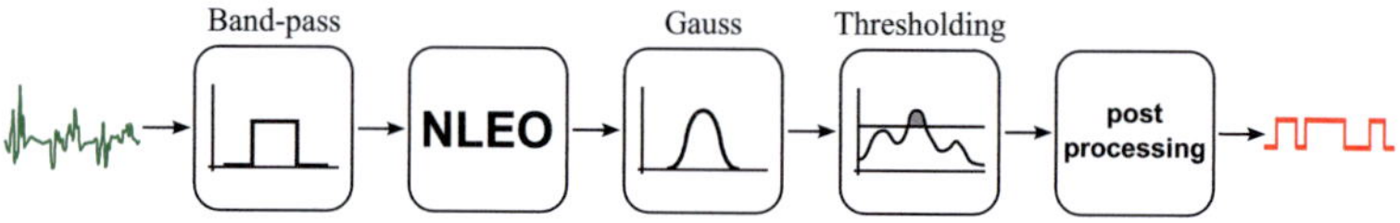

Fig. 6.6: Block diagram of the NLEO segmentation algorithm.

6.4 Results of CFAE Segmentation

The presented segmentation algorithm to find active segments in atrial electrograms is an important basis to reflect the physicians view on EGMs and the subsequent analysis of EGMs and CFAEs. Regularly, the baseline of CFAEs is unsteady and irregular. Also the amplitude of deflections is varying and there is no periodicity like during SR or AFlut. By use of the NLEO, both, frequency and amplitude are taken into account to measure a CFAE's dynamic. Parts with high frequency and/or large amplitude are detected and small deflections are suppressed by the low-pass filtered NLEO. The signal's dynamic can be detected and analyzed by use of an adaptive thresholding. In this way, large and low amplitudes as well as high and low frequency parts will be detected, even if they are in close proximity. Unlike methods based on the analysis of the signal frequency, perturbation of the baseline does not affect the result of our algorithm. The NLEO is mostly insensitive to baseline wander, as it is computed from just three adjacent values.

During endocardial mapping, CFAEs are in the focus of interest since they are associated with the AF substrate. In EGMs, sections with a prolonged activation complex are key indices for CFAEs. By defining a refractory period, CFAE sections can be identified in their total length. This is achieved by a postprocessing step, where adjacent active sections with a gap smaller than 42 ms are merged. Therefore, active segments in the segmented signal represent the electrophysiological activity (fig. 6.7).

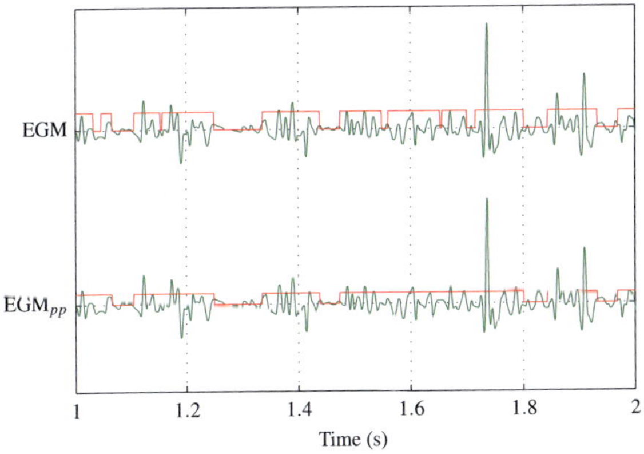

Fig. 6.7: Effect of post-processing the CFAE segmentation. Small gaps between active segments are ignored and adjacent active segments are merged. Active segments are marked with a red step function.

The advantage of the NLEO-based segmentation, compared e.g. with the CFAE-mean, is that this algorithm will also find segments of different length and therefore, reflect the physicians' view on CFAEs more naturally. Figure 6.8 depicts two signal parts of a CFAE recorded during atrial fibrillation. The EGM on the left hand side is segmented into active segments with different length, although the single segments have different amount of fractionation and different amplitudes. The EGM on the right hand side is segmented correctly, although the amplitudes are varying heavily.

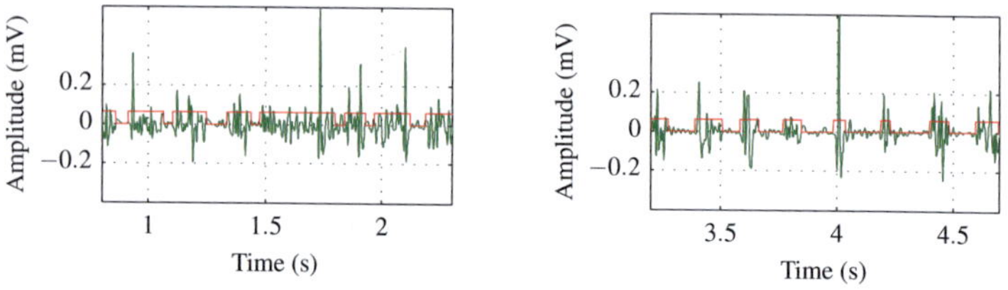

Fig. 6.8: CFAEs divided into active and inactive segments by use of the NLEO approach.

There is at the moment no public database for atrial electrograms and especially CFAEs. So, there is no public data with marked fiducial points that can be used as reference for testing the algorithm. Therefore, the evaluation of this algorithm was done qualitatively. Electrograms during different atrial rhythms have been recorded and the method was applied on the data. Finally, the segmented EGMs have been evaluated by physicians.

Data from 5 patients has been used for evaluation. The electrograms had a length of 5 seconds and were recorded during sinus rhythm, atrial flutter, and atrial fibrillation. Figure 6.9 depicts example electrograms for each rhythm. The red step function marks active and inactive segments. Segmentation works for all atrial rhythms and active segments are identified correctly. The NLEO-based segmentation of EGMs is the basis of analyzing CFAEs and to classify them. A set of descriptors will be defined on basis of the segmentation (chapter 7).

The NLEO-based segmentation could also be used to detect the QRS complex in the surface ECG. For this, parameters would have to be adjusted (average peak width, length of the time-window to calculate thresholds and refractory period) as the morphology of surface ECG components are different to atrial ones.

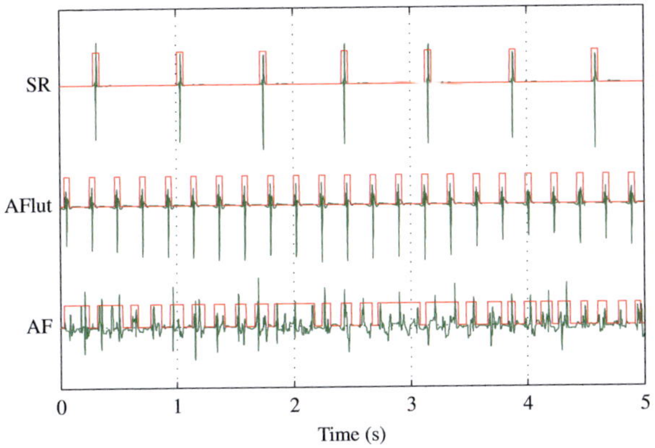

Fig. 6.9: EGM divided into active and inactive segments by use of the NLEO approach.

7

Describing Atrial Electrograms

Electrograms, especially CFAEs, tend to be very complex shaped signals. To characterize these kinds of signals a set of descriptors will be introduced in the following chapter. A descriptor is a number computed as describing feature of the electrogram. Descriptors will delineate the behavior of an electrogram's feature as well as give a measure for this feature. Before computing a descriptor of a signal, the signal is preprocessed as described in section 4.4.

7.1 Test and Evaluation of Descriptors

The descriptors will be evaluated on data measured during EP studies. To reflect the influence of the atrial rhythm evolving from sinus rhythm (SR) via atrial flutter (AFlut) to atrial fibrillation (AF) on the descriptors three example signals for each rhythm will be used (fig. 7.1).
The output of the descriptors is also evaluated on the different CFAE types occurring during AF (sec. 4.2.1). Therefore, four example signals (fig. 7.2) for each defined CFAE class will be used to reflect the distinction potential of a descriptor.
Some descriptors are only used to distinguish between contact and non contact catheter signals (chap. 9). Therefore, the outcome of these descriptors is shown on two electrograms representing a contact and a non-contact EGM (fig. 7.3).
Finally, to show also the statistical outcome of a descriptor's result, the distribution of descriptor values of the different CFAE classes will be shown as boxplot complemented with an estimated probability density distribution (appendix A). As basis for this evaluation the signals of the database presented in section 4.3.1 will be used.

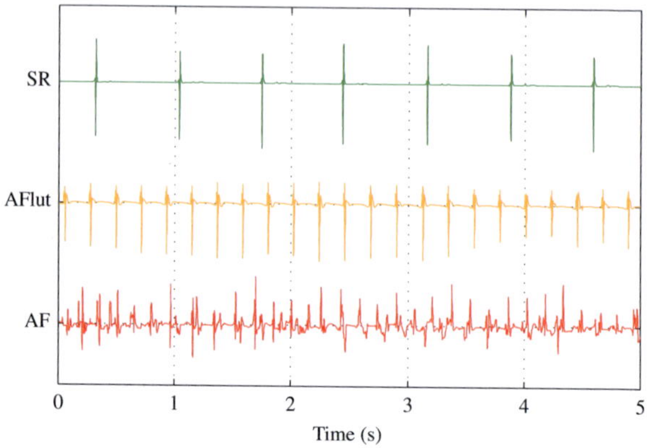

Fig. 7.1: Typical atrial signals during sinus rhythm, atrial flutter, and atrial fibrillation.

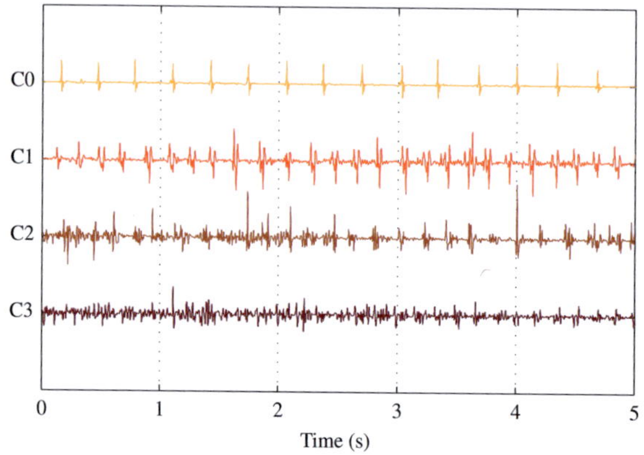

Fig. 7.2: Atrial example signals for the different CFAE classes occurring during atrial fibrillation.

7.2 Amplitude Statistics-based Descriptors

The excess is a statistical measure of the curvature of a probability density function. If the excess is calculated on the amplitude histogram of an electrogram it represents the amplitude distribution of this electrogram. Electrograms during sinus rhythm (fig. 7.1) contain only few areas with large amplitude alteration, whereas

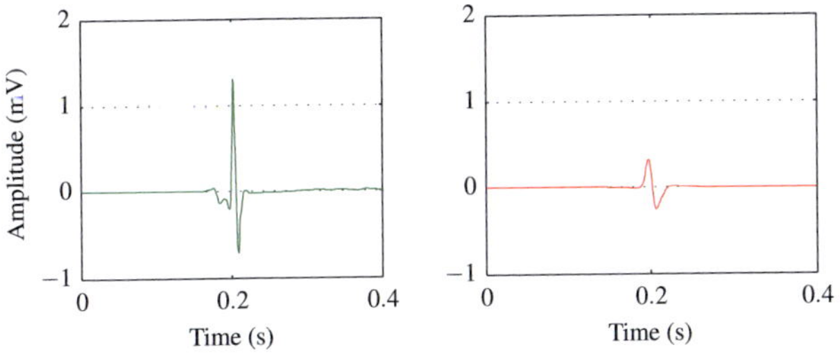

Fig. 7.3: Atrial example signals for contact (left) and non-contact signals (right).

in wide areas the amplitude is zero. This is reflected in a sharp peak and short tails in the histogram. The excess of these signals attains large values. CFAEs (fig. 7.2) instead are characterized by wide non-zero areas which will lead to a broad and flat distribution (more gaussian). The excess of CFAEs attains smaller values. If the distribution is a gaussian distribution the excess is zero. For even smaller and flatter distributions the excess attains negative values. To be robust against outliers,

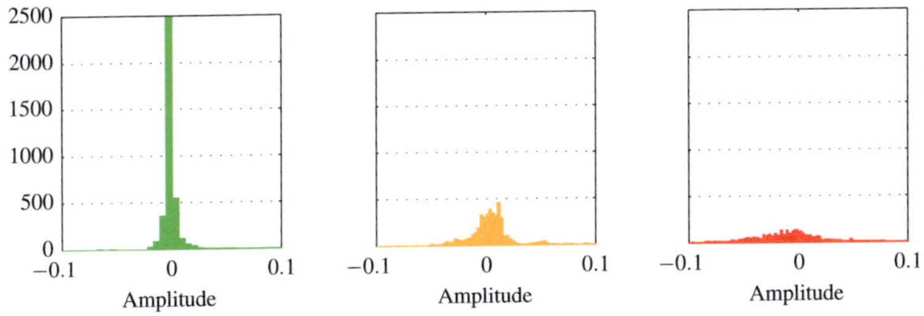

Fig. 7.4: Amplitude histogram for EGMs during sinus rhythm (left), atrial flutter (middle), and atrial fibrillation (right).

the electrogram is divided into 1 sec. segments. The segment length is chosen to 1 sec to have at least one beat per segment even during a heart frequency of 60 beats/sec. On each segment the excess is computed. The excess (HistExc) of a given electrogram then is the mean excess of all segments:

$$\text{HistExc} = \frac{1}{k}\sum_{j=0}^{k-1} \text{excess}(x(t|j \cdot 1\text{ sec} \leq t \leq (j+1) \cdot 1\text{ sec})) \tag{7.1}$$

To examine the signal curve within an active (AS), the low-pass filtered NLEO segment of an AS ($\mathrm{E_{NLEO}}$) will be interpreted as probability density function. Thus, statistic moments like the excess, kurtosis, or standard deviation can be computed. In this case the standard deviation will give a measure for the concentration of the signal curve in time direction. Therefore, the integral of a NLEO segment is normalized to 1 ($\tilde{\mathrm{E}}_{\mathrm{NLEO}}$) and the standard deviation in time direction is calculated. To be independent of the segment length, the standard deviation is divided by the length l of the AS

$$\sigma_{\tilde{\mathrm{E}}_{\mathrm{NLEO}}} = \sqrt{\sum_{i=1}^{l} (i - \mu_{\tilde{\mathrm{E}}_{\mathrm{NLEO}}})^2 \cdot \tilde{\mathrm{E}}_{\mathrm{NLEO,i}} / l}. \tag{7.2}$$

The mean variation in time domain (mVarTD) for an electrogram is computed as mean of the mVarTD values achieved from all AS within that electrogram. For regular signals the NLEO, and therefore its variation in time, is mainly symmetric and Gaussian-like. The more complex and high fractionated the signal curve of an AS is, the more variation will be found in the NLEO.

Table 7.1: Results of amplitude based descriptors applied on example data (fig. 7.1, 7.2).

	SR	AFlut	AF	C0	C1	C2	C3
HistExc	22.77	36.72	9.37	29.11	9.25	10.63	4.84
mVarTD	0.15	0.16	0.22	0.16	0.20	0.22	0.26

7.3 Time Domain Descriptors Based on NLEO

Based on the NLEO segmentation algorithm introduced in sec. 6.3 a set of descriptors can be defined. The sum of the length of all active segments during a 5 s recording divided by the total length of the signal is called activity ratio (AR)

$$\mathrm{AR} = \frac{1}{L} \sum_{i=1}^{n} l_i, \tag{7.3}$$

with L the length of the total signal, n the number of active segments and l_i the length of an active segment.

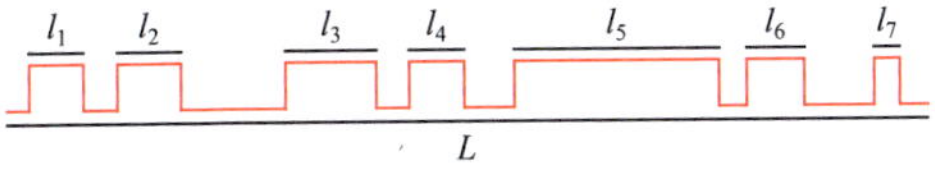

Fig. 7.5: Activity ratio.

Another descriptor is the mean length of active segments (MLAS), which is defined as

$$\mathrm{MLAS} = \frac{1}{n}\sum_{i=1}^{n} l_i \tag{7.4}$$

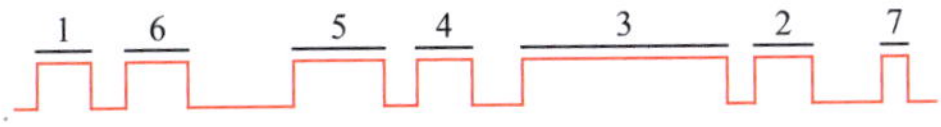

Fig. 7.6: Mean length of active segments.

The mean length of inactive segments (MLiAS) is defined analogically on the inactive segments. The standard deviation (SD) of active segments (SDAS) is defined as

$$\mathrm{SDAS} = \sqrt{\frac{1}{n}\sum_{i=1}^{n} (l_i - \mathrm{MLAS})^2} \tag{7.5}$$

Five more descriptors are defined based on the identified active segments. These are the number of active segments (NoAS), the mean number (ZCAS) and variance of zero crossings per active segment (varZCAS), and the mean number (LocMaxAS) and variance of local maxima per active segment (varMaxAS).
The numbers resulting from ZCAS, varZCAS, LocMaxAS, and varMaxAS are not linearly distributed. As these discriptors are also used to build a fuzzy decision tree, the descriptor values should be preferably distributed homogeneously. The decision function of a fuzzy decision tree is defined symmetrically around the split point. Therefore, to achieve more linearly distributed values, the natural logarithm is computed on these descriptors.

7.4 Similarity of Active Segments

With increasing fractionation of an electrogram the similarity of activation patterns is decreasing as well as the periodicity. Faes et. al. [120] described an algorithm that compares the similarity of different regions of an intracardiac signal. They

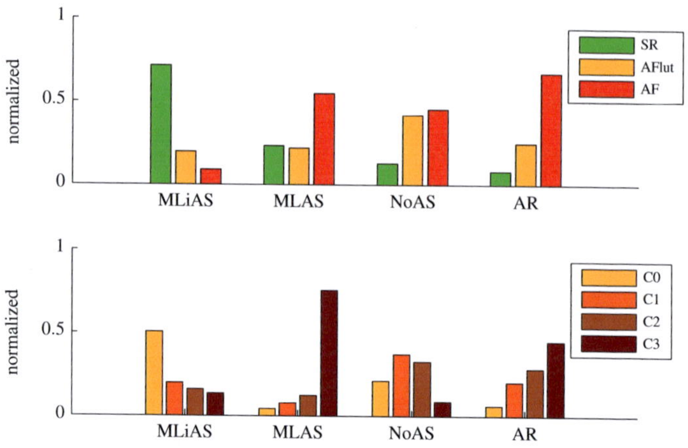

Fig. 7.7: Results of some NLEO-based descriptors.

Table 7.2: Results of NLEO-based descriptors applied on example data (fig. 7.1, 7.2).

	SR	AFlut	AF	C0	C1	C2	C3
MLiAS (ms)	578	160	71	325	128	103	88
MLAS (ms)	53	50	125	52	97	153	934
NoAS	7	23	25	15	26	23	6
AR	0.07	0.23	0.63	0.13	0.42	0.59	0.93
ZCAS	1.19	1.64	1.94	1.58	1.80	2.56	4.27
varZCAS	−1.44	−0.86	2.90	0.12	1.52	4.68	8.73
LocMaxAS	1.15	1.76	2.40	1.80	2.15	2.79	4.49
varMaxAS	−1.95	−0.13	3.79	−0.70	1.65	5.04	9.27

extracted segments with fixed windows around the activation patterns and made a clustering process on these segments to get a measure for their similarity. Inspired by Faes' work a new similarity analysis of CFAEs is computed. Therefore, the envelope of the absolute value of the analytical signal is calculated according to the algorithm described in [121]. The envelope follows the signal's shape, but is always positiv. The envelope is used because as the signal's fractionation is increasing the accurate shape is varying strongly, but the envelope reflects the general shape (fig. 7.8). Active segments within a signal are extracted with the

NLEO-based segmentation algorithm. Next, the analytical signal within the active segments is calculated.

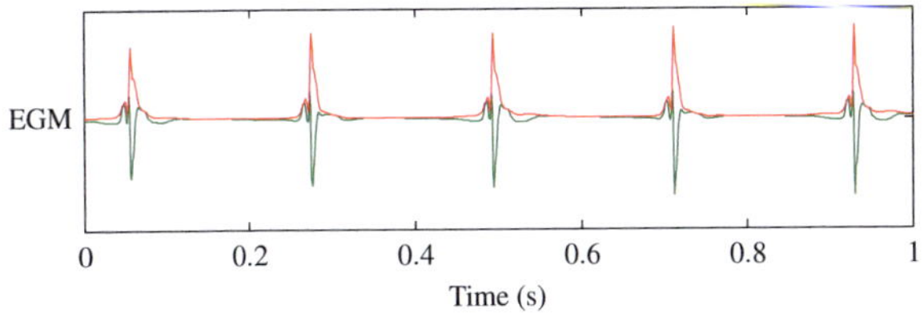

Fig. 7.8: Electrogram (green) with its analytical signal (red).

With these extracted segments a correlation matrix is built. First of all, the segments are aligned using cross correlation. Then, the absolute value of the correlation coefficient is calculated on the overlapping parts as similarity measure. Based on this correlation matrix a clustering is performed. Starting a cluster with the two most similar segments, step by step the nearest similar segment is added and the similarity between the new segment and the cluster is computed. The similarity of the cluster and the segment is computed with (7.6). Figure 7.9 depicts the similarity curves for the example CFAEs. According to the definition of Kaufmann and Rousseuw [122] the similarity between two clusters is calculated from

$$s(R,Q) = \frac{1}{|R||Q|} \sum_{i \in R, j \in Q} s(i,j) \tag{7.6}$$

$|R|$ and $|Q|$ are the cardinalities of both clusters, $s(i,j)$ is the similarity between element i from cluster R and the element j from cluster Q. Here, the number of elements of cluster Q is set to 1 (only one segment) and R is increasing by one with every new segment that is taken into account. Finally, the mean value of the similarities of a signal (fig. 7.9) is computed as descriptor.

7.5 Frequency Analysis of CFAEs, Periodicity Detection

7.5.1 CFAEmean

The fractionation index CFAEmean is an invention of St. Jude Medical and is used in their EnSite NavX™ system to analyze electrograms during an electrophysio-

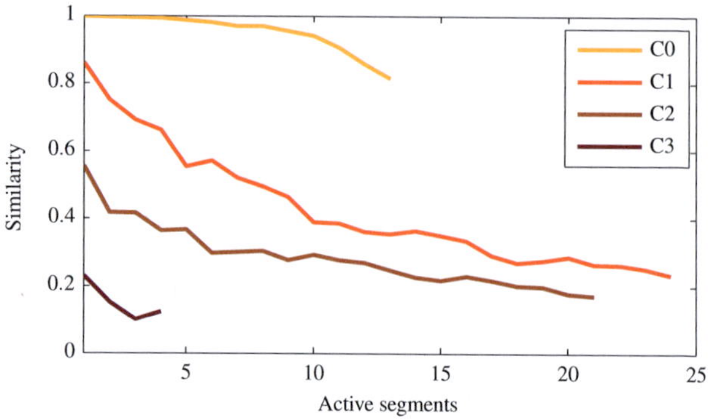

Fig. 7.9: Similarity of active segments of different CFAEs. For very similar segments the similarity attains values near 1.

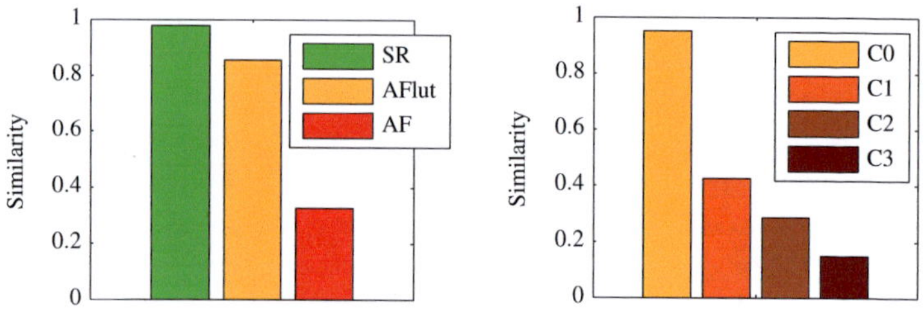

Fig. 7.10: Mean similarity of active segments for the example EGMS.

logical examination. There are a lot of parameters that can be set by the physician for the calculation of CFAEmean:

- Detection method (−dV/dt)
- Reference sensitivity (0.3)
- Minimal width (10 ms)
- Refractory period (42 ms)
- Segment length (5 s)
- Peak-peak sensitivity (0.04)

Values for a typical setup are given in brackets. The algorithm is very adjustable, but this is also a big disadvantage. As each physician has his/her own settings, the result of the CFAEmean is not comparable to other physicians' results. The CFAEmean index searches for a falling edge in the EGM fulfilling the sensitivity precept. This point is marked as begin of a fractionated electrogram complex with the assumed width of 10 ms and a refractory period of 42 ms. Then the beginning of the following fractionated complex is searched. This is done for the whole electrogram (5 sec). The mean distance between the found marks is defined as CFAEmean. The CFAEmean is based on the cycle length between discriminable local activities in the EGM (fig. 7.11).

$$\text{CFAEmean} = \text{mean cycle length of local activity}$$

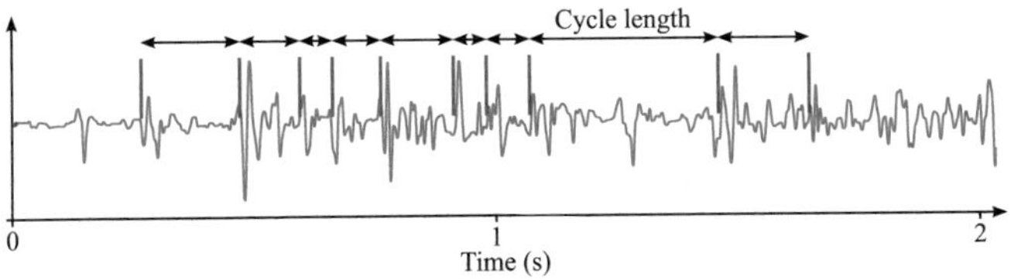

Fig. 7.11: CFAEmean algorithm developed by St. Jude Medical.

7.5.2 Dominant Frequency

To analyze EGMs or CFAEs in particular in the frequency domain, Everett et al. [119] proposed a method that transforms the envelope of a signal by use of the FFT. This algorithm is based on the envelope detection algorithm by Botteron and Smith [123]. After band-pass filtering with a passband of 40 Hz to 250 Hz, to accentuate the signal corresponding to the local depolarization, the filter's output is rectified and low-pass filtered with a cut-off frequency of 20 Hz. The band-pass filter is realized as a Generalized-Equiripple-Filter with $f_{\text{stop1}} = 35$ Hz, $f_{\text{pass1}} = 45$ Hz, $f_{\text{pass2}} = 250$ Hz , $f_{\text{stop2}} = 270$ Hz. The applied low-pass filter is realized as Generalized-Equiripple-Filter with $f_{\text{pass}} = 18$ Hz, $f_{\text{stop}} = 35$ Hz. The damping at the stop/pass frequencies is 40 dB. The lowpass filtering at 20 Hz limits the spectrum to frequencies that fall within a reasonable physiologic range of activation rates.

Before applying the FFT, windowing is a common maneuver to attenuate discontinuities at the beginning and end of a segment gradually to zero to reduce their effect on the spectrum. This is achieved by multiplying a rounded waveform, such as the Hanning or Kaiser window [83]. The resulting envelope is Fourier transformed. The power spectrum of an EGM regularly has a dominant peak in the frequency range 3 Hz to 20 Hz. The frequency according to this peak is called dominant frequency.

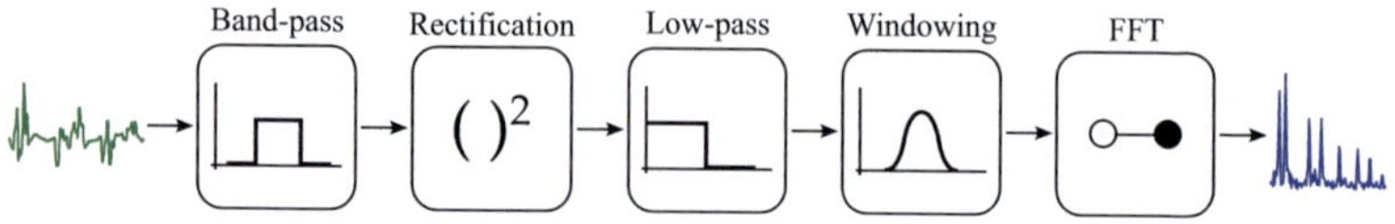

Fig. 7.12: Block diagram of the dominant frequency algorithm. The signal's envelope is Fourier transformed to reflect the atrial activation rate. The frequency peak with the highest amplitude is assumed to be the dominant frequency.

Everett et al. also examined the influence of the signal length on the result of the DF. They found that too short signals have not enough information to be analyzed with the DF. Also the frequency resolution of too short signals is not sufficient. Too long signals have a better frequency resolution, but they have also more intermediate peaks. Finding the dominant frequency will getting harder. According to Everett a signal length of 4 seconds works best for analysis with DF [119].
DF approximates the atrial activation rate. DF works better, the more the signal's envelope looks like a sinusoidal. This implies that DF will only find one activation rate per signal. As long as the deflections of the EGM are regular equidistant, DF is a robust and effective tool to approximate the activation rate. For very complex signals like CFAEs, where the atrial activation is more chaotic, non-regular, and parts of continuous activity are present, a mean activation rate does not make sense at all. These signals can also be interpreted as a superimposition of different activation processes and DF will not reflect this behavior [124, 125].

7.5.3 Characteristic Frequencies

As mentioned in the previous section the DF will fail if the EGM is a result of superimposed activation processes. From this premiss analyzing only a single frequency will loose significant information. Hence, it is promising to search not only for the most prominent frequency in the EGM's spectrum, but search also for the second and third prominent frequency. These frequencies will be called characteristic frequencies (CF). Similar to the DF analysis, first of all, the EGM's envelope is computed. After a Fourier transform the CF is determined. In contrast to the envelope detection method used for the computation of the DF (sec. 7.5.2) the low-pass filtered NLEO of the EGM is used. The NLEO's output is not only proportional to the amplitude of the EGM, but also to the EGM's frequency (sec. 6.2). Small alterations of the isoelectric line will be suppressed better by the NLEO. So, segments of different activity can be better differentiated. Figure 7.13 depicts the output of the envelope method by Everett [119] compared to the low-pass filtered NLEO of the shown EGM.

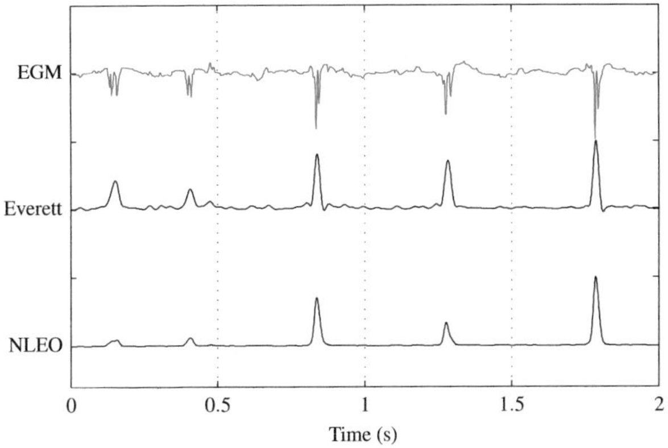

Fig. 7.13: Envelope detection of EGMs. Comparison of the method by Everett [119] and the low-pass filtered NLEO.

The frequency rate of atrial fibrillation is between 4 – 10 Hz, which corresponds to 240 – 600 beats per minute [1, 3]. So the range in which CF can occur is also between 4 and 10 Hz. On order to not only detect the frequencies with the most prominent amplitude in the spectrum but also the frequencies that have fundamental meaning to the EGM, only frequency peaks with dominant harmonics are considered as candidates for CF. Looking only at the first harmonic would put strong weight on a small sinusoidal signal and small weight on strong signals that show up regularly but do not have a sinusoidal shape. The algorithm proposed in this thesis takes the first three harmonics into account. This extends the interesting frequency range to 4 – 40 Hz. The most prominent peak with the smallest frequency in the range 4 – 10 Hz is taken and its harmonics are searched in the remaining peaks up to 40 Hz. If harmonics are found, this frequency is a candidate for a CF. The procedure is repeated for all prominent peaks in the range 4 – 10 Hz.

Commonly, an envelope of a CFAE will result in very irregular PDS distributions. Thus, a lot of CFs will be found, that match the definition of a CF, but do not have physiological meaning. Also, the frequency of a cardiac excitation can change slowly over time. In consequence, the spectrum may contain a number of CFs with close proximity to each other. Hence, some restrictions are defined to detect wrong CFs.

- According to the maximal CF peak all further CFs must be prominent. That means, that all further CFs must have a peak that is at least half of the maximal CF peak.
- The distance between two adjacent CF peaks must be at least 0.25 Hz.
- A CF must not be a multiple of a previous CF, otherwise it might be itself a harmonic of the previous CF.

When deleting a CF because of these restrictions, the stronger of the two frequencies, i.e. the frequency with the greater peak, is kept. Thus, all meaningful CFs in the frequency band of 4 – 10 Hz will be detected.
Figure 7.14 depicts an AFlut and an AF signal with their PDS and the found CFs. For AFlut there is only one characteristic frequency (4.5 Hz), whereas three CFs are found for the AF case (tab. 7.3). Table 7.3 also shows the case of SR. There is an obvious difference in the PDS, too. The PDS of the AFlut signal looks regular and the CF with its harmonics is distinctly to recognize. The PDS of the AF signal is more irregular and prominent peaks are not as easy to recognize.
From this observation, the area under each CF in a frequency band of ± 0.5 Hz in ratio to the area of the bandwidth 4 – 10 Hz seems to be a good measure to separate the different rhythms. For regular signals the area under a CF will be much larger, than for continuous activity.

Table 7.3: Results of CF applied on EGMs during SR, AFlut, and AF.

	CF1	CF2	CF3
SR	1.4 Hz	–	–
AFlut	4.5 Hz	–	–
AF	1.8 Hz	6.3 Hz	6.8 Hz

After detecting characteristic frequencies, these can be transposed onto the time signal of the NLEO. Assuming that active segments can contain signal contents

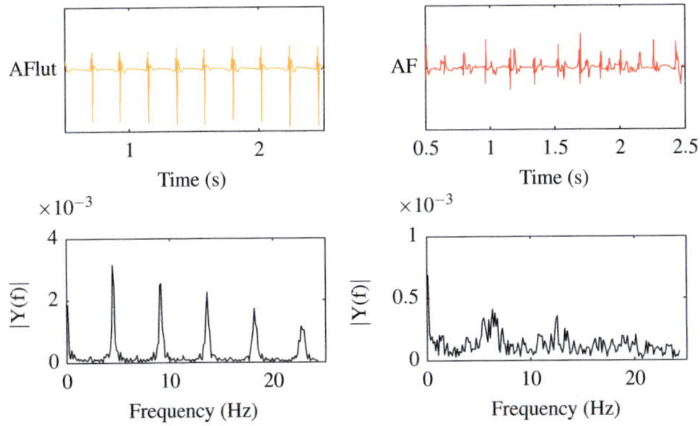

Fig. 7.14: On the left hand side an atrial flutter signal with its PDS is shown. On the right hand side an atrial fibrillation signal with its PDS is depicted. The PDS is calculated on the output of the NLEO. There is an distinct difference in the PDS representation.

from different triggers, the NLEO found in an active segment will be a superimposition of the NLEO of these triggers.The NLEO-based segmentation method, combines active segments, when the gap between them is smaller than 42 ms. This holds true, when detecting atrial activity. For this purpose, where signal parts are assumed to belong to different CFs, it is feasible to partition the active segment into multiple subsegments based on an extremum criterion. The NLEO curve will be divided into segments at a minimum falling in between two maxima. Figure 7.15 shows a typical case where two NLEO activity patterns are merged, because of a short lag. The signal will be divided into two segments at its minimum.

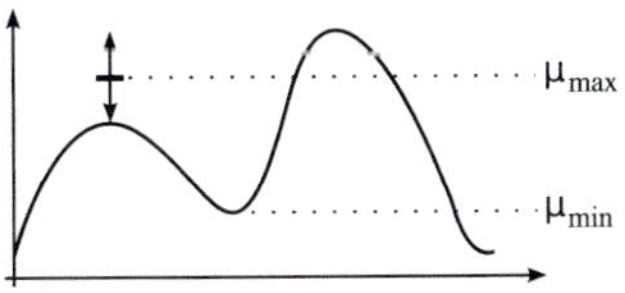

Fig. 7.15: Reshaping active segments.

All extreme values in the NLEO are searched. Only minima that fall in between two maxima are candidates for a split point. The minima at the beginning or the ending of a segment are discarded. Out of the remaining extreme values, the mean minimum and the mean maximum value are calculated. The segment will be cut apart, when the found minimum is smaller than 90% of the mean maximum. This threshold is chosen, to ensure, that the minimum is significantly different from a maximum. Otherwise this minimum could also be a noisy deflection and is no candidate for splitting. After cutting the active segments apart, new segments with very small activity (NLEO values) might be found. These segments reflect rather noise than atrial activity. Therefore, all new segments, whose peak is smaller than 5% of the maximum peak of the original segment, will be discarded. Figure 7.16 gives an example of the NLEO's segmentation before and after applying the proposed algorithm.

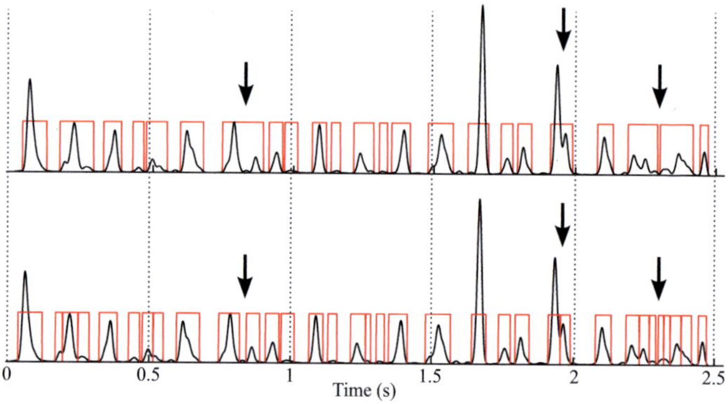

Fig. 7.16: Example of the reshaping process applied on the NLEO of an electrogram. The upper figure depicts the segmenting before and the lower figure after reshaping.

For each CF an according cycle length can be computed. Based on this cycle length, segments should be found, that have the same distinct spacing. Therefore, each segment will be represented by a prominent point to find these recurring spacings. To determine the most prominent point of a segment, finding its NLEO maximum might be a good choice. However, this may be misleading, when the NLEO is asymmetric. Instead of the NLEO's maximum peak, the center of gravity for this segment is calculated. Starting with the first center of gravity, the subsequent is supposed in a spacing according to the CF. So, beginning with the first segment and its respective center of gravity for the following segments, it is checked, if

there is a center of gravity in the spacing of the corresponding cycle length. If this holds true, the AS segment is marked as positive match; if not, the AS is marked as negative match. This is repeated until all segments are processed or there are two negative matches in a sequence. When the first row of detection is finished or aborted, the procedure is repeated starting from the second segment. This procedure is done until the algorithm has been started from all segments. As result multiple combs of detection, with positive and negative matches, are obtained for each CF. Some combs might be a subset of others, caused by successively starting a comb of detection at each segment. Subsets that overlap for the same segments are merged. Also, subsets are concatenated, when the last positive match of the first comb and the first match of the second comb belong to the same segment. This procedure is done for all detected CFs.
The latter method of transposing the CFs back into time domain will not lead to a special descriptor, but will give a new perspective on complex fractionated atrial electrograms. Thus, it will help understanding the origin of CFAEs and the different types of CFAEs or complex atrial rhythms. Figure 7.17 depicts the results of this method on a CFAE. The original CFAE and the original NLEO-based segmentation is shown in the upper graph. Whereas, the lower graph depicts the NLEO and its new segmentation. In both graphs the found comb of detections for three CFs are shown. For this CFAE there is a base frequency of 6.01 Hz being present in the whole signal. Whereas, the frequencies of 7.17 Hz and 4.58 Hz are occurring and vanishing over time. This could be, for example, caused by a rotor as trigger for these frequencies.
A second example (fig. 7.18) was recorded during sinus rhythm. A slowly changing frequency in the signal can be seen. The red, green, and black combs represent 1.07, 1.11, and 1.15 Hz. This kind of analysis can, therefore, be used during catheter ablation, when monitoring the change of the cycle length (or frequency) of the arrhythmia.

7.5.4 Power Density Spectrum-based Descriptors

When loosing catheter contact to the endocardium electrograms are getting dull and the amplitude is decreasing. This is caused by vanishing high frequency components of the electrogram [126]. Figure 7.19 shows this circumstance. The lower pictures show the power density spectrum (PDS) of the signals shown in the upper line. The bandwidth is nearly halved comparing contact to non-contact EGM.

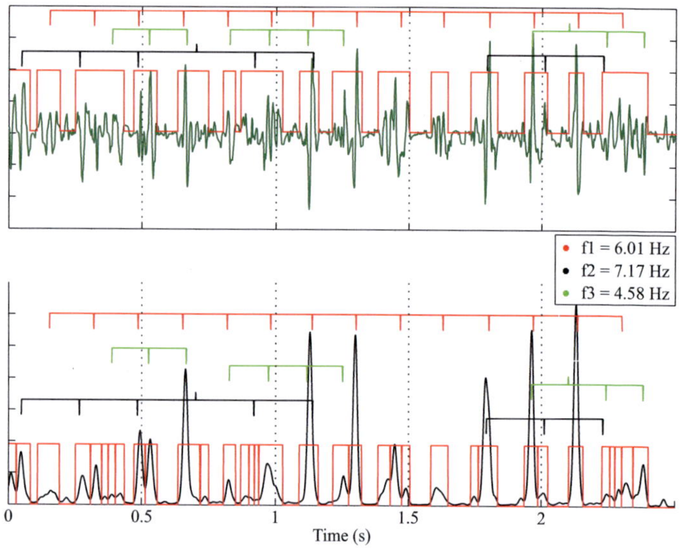

Fig. 7.17: Periodicity detection in case of atrial fibrillation.

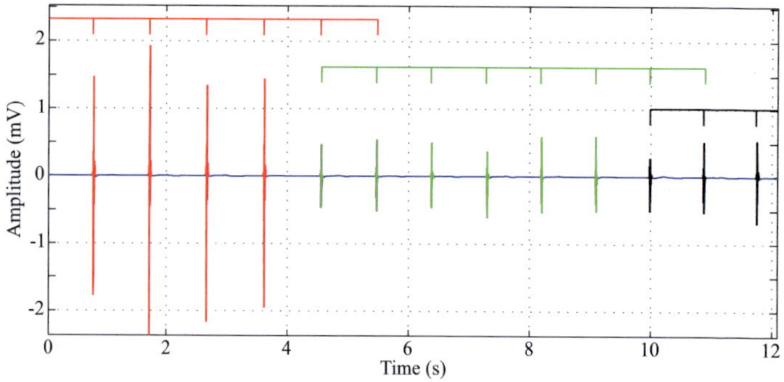

Fig. 7.18: Periodicity detection during sinus rhythm with a slow changing frequency. The red comb represents 1.07 Hz, the green comb 1.11 Hz, and the black comb 1.15 Hz.

Thus, analyzing the power density spectrum will be helpful when dividing contact from non-contact EGMs. The main frequency content for EGMs will be found beneath a threshold of 200 Hz. The area from 0 – 200 Hz is normalized to be independent from a signal's amplitude. Then, the area beneath the PDS curve between

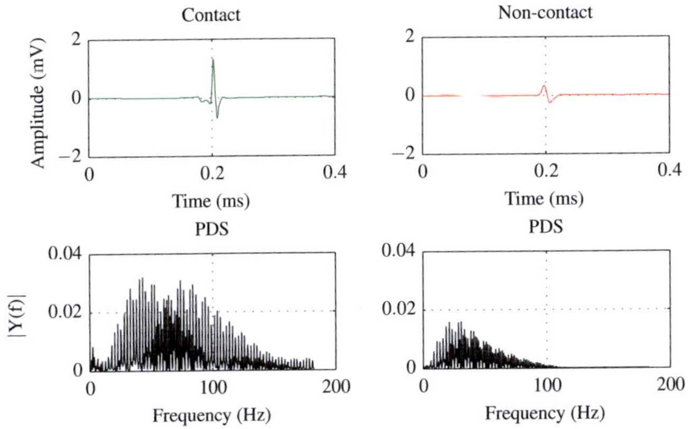

Fig. 7.19: Comparison of the power density spectrum of a contact and a non-contact EGM.

0 – 90 Hz is computed. The percental frequency distribution in this area is defined as descriptor. Contact EGMs are expected to result in smaller values as they have a broader frequency distribution over the complete range than non-contact EGMs. A similar descriptor is defined for the frequency range 130 – 300 Hz as in this range no non-contact signal frequency is expected. Another descriptor to measure the different distributions is the amplitude of the first peak after 100 Hz. For contact signals this will result in larger values than for non-contact signals. The envelope of the frequency distributions from 0 – 200 Hz is computed, normalized to 1, and interpreted as density function. So, central moments (like excess and skewness) can be derived as descriptors. Central moments describe the shape of the frequency distribution.

7.6 PCA-based Descriptors

The signals of the contact/non-contact database (sec. 4.3.3) are aligned to their maximum and a data vector of signals is created. When applying a PCA on this vector, the signals related to one class are located in one area of the PCA space. These regions can be separated by a thresholding. According to this threshold a new signal can be allocated to a region and therefore to one class. Based on the first principle component a hard threshold is defined, so that the distance to the

Table 7.4: Results of PDS based descriptors applied on example data (fig. 7.19).

	contact	non-contact
Percental frequency distribution 0 – 90 Hz	68%	96%
Percental frequency distribution 130 – 300 Hz	2.2%	0%
Max. energy peak < 100 Hz	40.48	1.67
Expectation value PDS envelope	280.42	142.47
Variance value PDS envelope	15 285	5794
Skewness value PDS envelope	0.76	2.04
Excess value PDS envelope	0.89	7.66

first score of each class is maximal. For a new, unknown signal the PCA score is calculated and an assignment to one class is made.
Examining the morphology of the first principle component gives a measure for the maximal variance in the data. Now applying a PCA only on contact signals will result in a characteristic variance for these signals. The same holds true for non-contact signals. Correlating a contact signal with the first PC gained from the contact class will result in larger correlation coefficients then computing the correlation coefficient with the first PC gained from non-contact signals.

Table 7.5: Results of PCA-based descriptors applied on example data (fig. 7.19).

	contact	non-contact
PCA-based decision	1.00	−0.50
Correlation with 1. PC non-contact	0.77	0.89
Correlation with 1. PC contact	0.87	0.68

7.7 Wavelet-based Descriptors

Kim & Kim [127] presented a method to detect action potentials in very noisy electroencephalograms by use of wavelet transform. With their algorithm it is possible to emphasize ranges of high slew rate within a signal. In the following section this algorithm is adapted for use with CFAEs to detect high fractionated ranges within an electrogram.
The electrogram is decomposed with Coiflet 4 into details and approximation up to level 10. Sharp peaks within an electrogram will result in a broad frequency range

in the frequency domain. Therefore, these peaks are represented in different detail levels as well. The detail level with the maximal occurring amplitude is searched. This level represents the most prominent content of the decomposed electrogram. The decomposition of an example electrogram is depicted in figure 7.20. Only the first six detail levels are displayed. Next, this level is point-wise multiplied with its two preceding (higher frequent) levels to emphasize high frequency content. Segments with high activity will be emphasized in the resulting representation of the electrogram, whereas segments with low activity will be suppressed. Figure 7.21 depicts the original electrogram and the resulting representation x_{res}

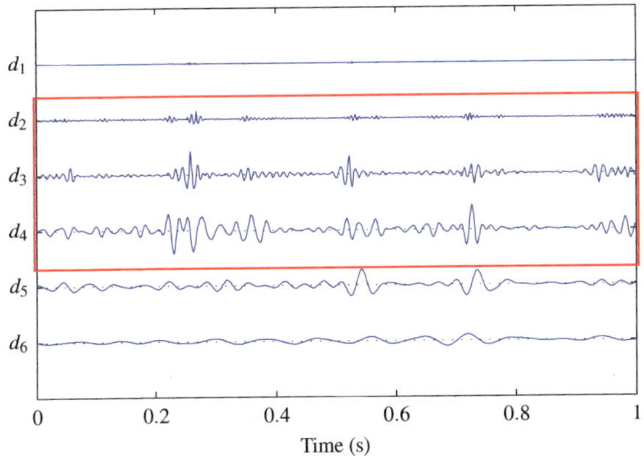

Fig. 7.20: Wavelet decomposition of example CFAE C2 with Coiflet 4. Level d4 is the level with the maximal amplitude and will be multiplied point-wise with the two preceding levels (red rectangle). Displayed is only the first second of the signal's decomposition.

after the described transposing method. Inactive segments in the electrogram are suppressed and well-nigh zero. In the remaining segments fractionated parts of the signal will be found by detection of zero-crossings. All zero-crossings above a threshold $x_{th} = 0.01 \cdot \sigma(x_{res})$ will be detected, with the standard deviation σ. Displaying the found zero-crossings on the electrogram shows that they correspond with active segments in the electrogram. Thus, the number of found zero-crossings can be used as measure for the fractionation of a given segment or electrogram.

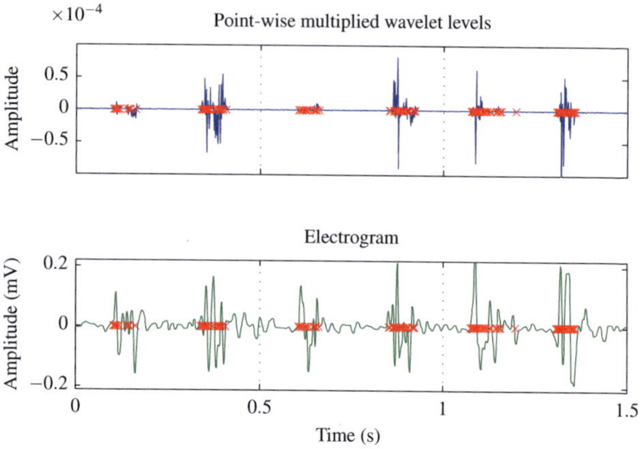

Fig. 7.21: Wavelet-based fractionation. The upper image depicts the point-wise multiplied wavelet levels found by the algorithm of [127]. The lower image depicts the original CFAE and the found fractionated areas (red crosses).

7.8 Phase Space-based Descriptors

A combined view of the signal's magnitude and the alteration at a position t_i is enabled by the phase space. Here, the signal's alteration $x'(t_i)$ is plotted over its magnitude $x(t_i)$. To weight the alteration and the magnitude equally, both are normalized to their maximum.

To analyze the distribution of the samples in phase space, the phase space is divided into circular regions. Therefore a maximal distance $d_{\max}$ to the point of origin is defined. The distance is calculated by

$$d(t_i) = \sqrt{x'(t_i)^2 + x(t_i)^2}. \tag{7.7}$$

To be more robust against outliers $d_{\max}$ is defined as the mean of 5% of the maximal distances $d_{0.05\max}$

$$d_{\max} = \frac{1}{0.05N} \sum_{j \in S} d(t_j), \quad \text{with } S = \{i | d(t_i) \in d_{0.05\max}\}. \tag{7.8}$$

Regular and periodical electrograms to large extent have values near zero and only a few large deflections that are non-zero (fig. 2.7). Most samples of these signals will be found in close proximity to the point of origin of the phase space. The more the electrogram gets fractionated, the less an isoelectric line is visible. These electrograms are characterized by a lot more deflections. The samples of these fractionated electrograms will be found preferentially in the outer regions of the phase space. Taking this into account the phase space is divided up into 4 regions depending on the distance d_{max}. Region 1 (magenta) encloses all sample values within a distance of 0.05 d_{max}. The border for region 2 (red) is at 0.1 d_{max}, for region 3 (green) at 0.2 d_{max}, and for region 4 (blue) at d_{max} (fig. 7.22). The number of samples in each region divided by the total number of samples is called phase space sample ratio (PSSR 1 magenta, PSSR 2 red, PSSR 3 green, PSSR 4 blue). Periodic signals, such as sinus rhythm electrograms, reach, for example,

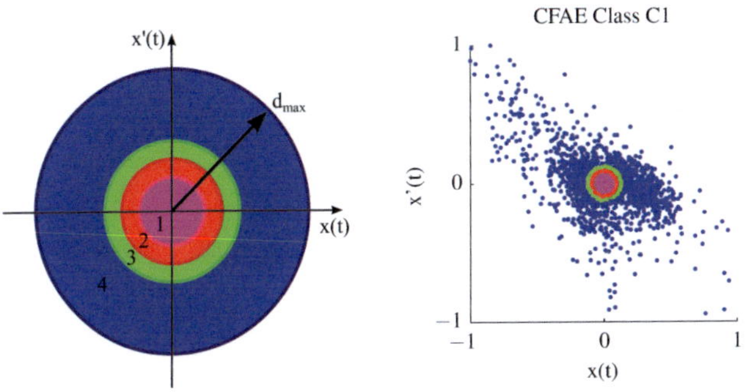

Fig. 7.22: Schematic representation of the 4 different regions in the phase space (left). On the right hand side a phase space example distribution of a CFAE class C1 signal is depicted.

the blue region (region 4) regularly. Chaotic or non-periodic signals do reach this blue region more randomly. To reflect this behavior a binary function is generated. This binary function equals '1', if a sample is located in the blue region, and '0' otherwise.

As the entropy mirrors the information content of a random process, the entropy is suitable to measure the periodicity of this binary function. The entropy of the binary function is termed as entropy of phase space (EPS) and is calculated for each region. To evaluate the periodicity of the binary function, the standard deviation of distances between two adjacent rising edges is calculated. The resulting descriptor is called mean cycle length of phase space (MCPS).

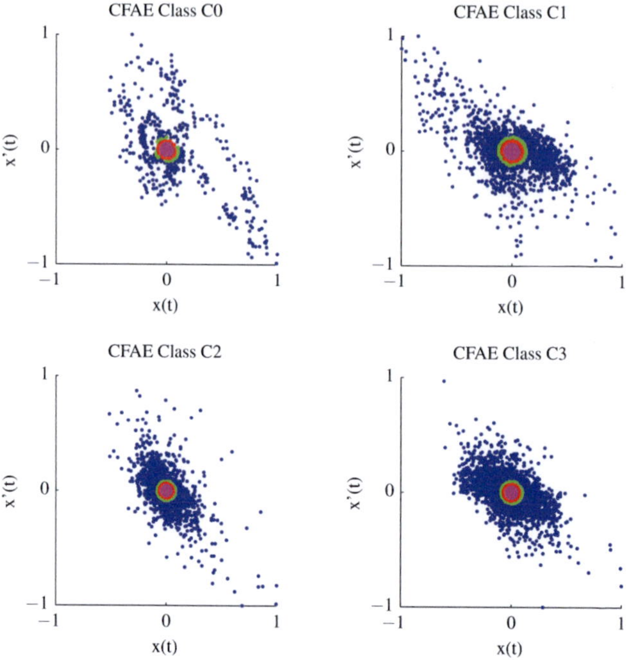

Fig. 7.23: An example of the phase space representation of different CFAE classes.

Figure 7.23 depicts the phase space distribution for the example CFAE signals. It can be seen, that fractionated signals (C1, C2, and C3) have a larger sample distribution in region 4 than C0. To evaluate the number of samples per region, figure 7.24 depicts a bar graph with the normalized number of samples per region. The number of samples of C0 is largest in region 1 and is decreasing over region 2 and 3 to region 4. The number of samples of C3 per region behaves the other way around. The samples of C1 and C2 are mostly scattered over region 2, 3, and 4. This was expected as regular signals have only few deflections, wheres fractionated signals have a lot more deflections. The results are summarized in table 7.6.

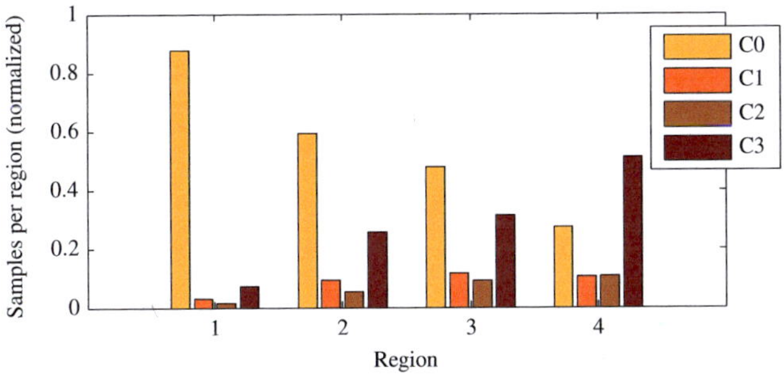

Fig. 7.24: Phase space sample ratio (PSSR) partitioned per CFAE class.

Table 7.6: Results of phase space-based descriptors applied on example data (fig. 7.1, 7.2).

	SR	AFlut	AF	C0	C1	C2	C3
PSSR 1	0.965	0.833	0.473	0.878	0.596	0.481	0.275
PSSR 2	0.004	0.050	0.133	0.032	0.093	0.113	0.104
PSSR 3	0.003	0.015	0.105	0.016	0.053	0.092	0.109
PSSR 4	0.028	0.103	0.289	0.074	0.258	0.313	0.512
EPS 4	1.20	1.64	2.63	1.55	2.46	2.69	2.50
MCPS 4	2.43	4.52	4.10	4.32	4.31	4.34	4.14

7.9 Results of Descriptors for EGMs

The presented descriptors can all be used to delineate and measure different features or attributes of atrial electrograms. Some descriptors delineate universal features of an EGM and others are used only for one special task (e.g. divide contact from non contact signals). An evaluation for all descriptors has been made with their introduction in the preceding sections. A more detailed view will also be taken, when using the descriptors in the following chapters. The descriptors are used to divide CFAEs into different classes, to separate contact from non-contact EGMs, or to generate new informations on EGMs recorded during catheter ablation.

The results of the descriptors used to classify CFAEs can be found in table 8.4 and in appendix A.1. Results and boxplots of the descriptors used to separate contact from non-contact signals can be found in table 9.2 and appendix A.2. Results of descriptors used for clinical trials can be found in part III.

8

Fuzzy Decision Tree to Classify CFAEs

Different types of CFAEs play a different role during ablation of AF. While ablating the physician classifies EGMs on the fly and decides whether an EGM is important for the ablation process or not. This decision is dependent on the personal experience of the physician. It would be a step towards objective signal analysis in the EP lab, when this classification process could be mirrored by an objective classifier. The classification by a physician is based on the experience of the physician as well as the history of a signal while ablation. Together with the physicians from Städtisches Klinikum Karlsruhe three typical classes of CFAEs (sec. 4.2.1) that occur during AF have been extracted. Sometimes CFAEs are measured, that do not obviously belong to one class. Often these CFAEs are classified to one or another class, depending on the physician's judgement. Besides the great experience in the field of ablating CFAEs, there is still an uncertainty in the classification of CFAEs. This implies, that there is also an uncertainty in the database of classified CFAEs included. Taking this into account, pure classification of an unknown signal by a decision tree could be ambiguous.
The combination of decision trees and fuzzy-logic combines classification with a probability estimation of the result. As result for each signal applied to the fuzzy decision tree a classification and a measure of certainty of the result is given. So, the reliability of a classification can be estimated.

8.1 Building the Fuzzy Decision Tree

The principles of decision making with a decision tree are introduced in section 3.8. One of the main shortcomings of decision trees with sharp split points is the result's sensitivity/vulnerability against small changes of the descriptor's value [128]. To overcome this problem, combining decision trees with fuzzy logic is a method proposed recently [129]. To obtain a fuzzy decision tree, it is possible to transpose the attributes in fuzzy-logic before building a regular decision tree. Another possibility is to build a regular tree and transpose the achieved decisions into fuzzy-logic [128].

The method to achieve fuzzy decision trees introduced in this section does not use sharp split points to separate classes, instead it uses a fuzzy zone to separate classes. According to the position in that fuzzy zone a test object will be assigned to one class with a specific probability. Thus, it is possible to assign objects in a region around the split point a relative affiliation to the following child nodes. This fuzzy zone is realized with a sigmoid function. The advantage of choosing a sigmoid function to make a fuzzy decision against other possible functions is, that the total affiliation of an attribute to the child nodes will always be 1. Sigmoid functions of form

$$\begin{aligned} z_l(k) &= 1 - \frac{1}{1+\exp\{-\sigma(a_k - s)\}} \\ z_r(k) &= \frac{1}{1+\exp\{-\sigma(a_k - s)\}} \end{aligned} \tag{8.1}$$

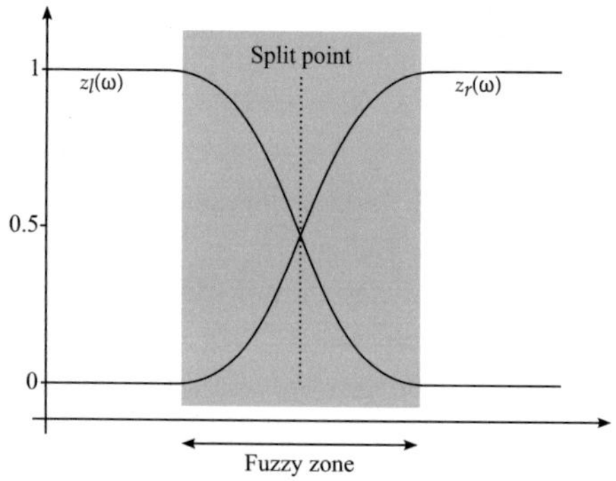

Fig. 8.1: Fuzzy decision process with a sigmoid function.

are proposed (fig. 8.1). z_l and z_r are the affiliation to the left and the right child node, s is the split point and a_k is the descriptor value of descriptor k. The coefficient σ is the standard deviation of this descriptor on the training data. If the descriptor values are scaled with a factor η, the width of the fuzzy zone is changing with η^2. This is not intended. Therefore a coefficient δ is defined to replace σ. The beginning z_{start} of the fuzzy zone is set when the sigmoid function equals 0.01 and the end z_{end} is set when the sigmoid function equals 0.99. In general $z_{start}(x) = g$ and $z_{end}(x) = 1 - g$. The range of a descriptor is the interval $[a_{k,\min}, a_{k,\max}]$. The width of the fuzzy zone is chosen as part $p \in [0,1]$ of the interval length $i = a_{k,\max} - a_{k,\min}$. It is assumed that the fuzzy zone with width $p \cdot i$ is set symmetrically to the split point s (fig. 8.1). This leads to

$$\begin{aligned} z_{start}(s - \frac{p \cdot i}{2}) &\stackrel{!}{=} g, \text{ and} \\ z_{end}(s + \frac{p \cdot i}{2}) &\stackrel{!}{=} 1 - g. \end{aligned} \tag{8.2}$$

The sigmoid function then is

$$z(x) = \frac{1}{1 + \exp\{-\delta(s - x)\}}. \tag{8.3}$$

Inserting (8.2) in (8.3) and solving for δ results in

$$\begin{aligned} \delta_1 &= -\frac{\ln(g) - \ln(1-g)}{-(p \cdot i)/2} \\ \delta_2 &= \frac{\ln(g) - \ln(1-g)}{(p \cdot i)/2}. \end{aligned} \tag{8.4}$$

With $\delta_1 = \delta_2$ one has

$$\delta = \frac{2(\ln(1-g) - \ln(g))}{p \cdot i}. \tag{8.5}$$

The boundaries for the interval $[a_{k,\min}, a_{k,\max}]$ have to be determined from the training data. To be robust against outliers, the upper boundary value is set to 1.5 interquartile range of the upper quartile and the lower boundary to 1.5 interquartile range of the lower quartile.

While training the decision tree it is the aim to find a split point at a node n_i, so that the relative membership of the objects to the right class is increasing. The Gini-Diversity-Index (GDI) is a regular criterion to evaluate possible split points [91]. Chandra et al. [128] presented an adaption of the GDI for usage in a fuzzy decision tree:

$$\mathrm{GDI}(s_m) = \sum_{v=1}^{2} \frac{N^{(t_v)}}{N^{(t)}} \cdot \left[1 - \sum_{m=1}^{M} \left(\frac{N_m^{(t_v)}}{N^{(t_v)}}\right)^2\right], \tag{8.6}$$

where M is the number of classes; $N^{(t_v)}$ is the sum of the fuzzy-membership values of records of child node t_v with chosen split point s_m on class m. $N^{(t)}$ is the sum of the fuzzy-membership values of records in the tth partition before splitting. $N_m^{(t_v)}$ is the sum of the product of fuzzy-membership values of the attribute and the fuzzy-membership values of the corresponding record for class m. For each descriptor vector the split point candidates are found and the candidate with the smallest GDI is chosen as split point.

While training a fuzzy decision tree the parameter p has to be set to define the width of the fuzzy zone. The distribution of classes within a descriptor distribution can differ. Thus, it might be advisable to choose an adjusted width for each descriptor. If there is a large overlap, the fuzzy zone should be larger than in the case of strictly separated classes. An approach to optimize the width of the fuzzy zone is to use the sensitivity of the GDI against the overlap of classes. For each split point the width of the fuzzy zone is optimized so that the GDI is minimal. This optimization is done by a combination of golden section search and a parabolic approximation to find a local minimum in a given range [130]. This optimization always leads to narrow fuzzy zones, independent of the class distribution. So, in the scope of this work, the best width of the fuzzy zone was determined by choosing the best result from a set of different fuzzy zones (fig. 8.2). For each fuzzy zone a 10×10 cross validation was realized and the mean error rate for the fuzzy zone was computed. Starting with a fuzzy width of 0%, the width was increased by 5% steps until reaching 50%. An additional sample was calculated for 2.5%. From 50% on, the step size was increased to 10%. The best error rate was achieved for a fuzzy zone width of 20%.

To make a decision on the class belonging of a given record, the decision tree needs an inference instruction. In contrast to a decision tree with sharp split values, where a record will get the class membership of the leaf node to which it is assigned, here, a test record can be assigned to more than one leaf node by a fuzzy decision tree. The inference instruction for a given record X_{Test} considers the fuzzy membership to a leaf node $z(n_i, X_{\mathrm{Test}})$ and its class membership $c(n_i)$. The fuzzy membership of a leaf node results from the product of fuzzy memberships of the passed nodes. The total class membership of a record X_{Test} is defined as

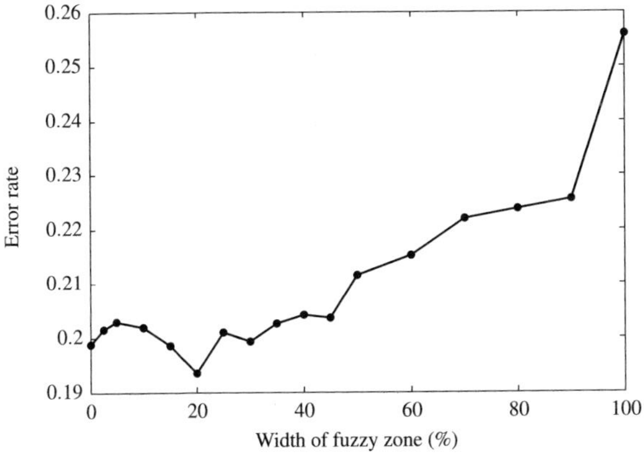

Fig. 8.2: Evaluation of different fuzzy zone widths to find the "best" fuzzy zone width. Displayed is the error rate as result of a 10×10 cross validation for each width.

$$c_{\text{total}}(X_{\text{Test}}) = \sum_i c(n_i) \cdot z(n_i, X_{\text{Test}}) \tag{8.7}$$

The classification of a record results in partial memberships to the classes. From these partial memberships the resulting class membership is derived by majority decision. The classified record will get the class label of the class with the highest membership percentage.

8.2 Pruning the Tree

Chandra et al. used different sharp stop criteria to limit the growth of the tree while training [128]. Stopping the tree growth during training phase is not the best way to limit tree size. Therefore, stop criteria are defined very weak to get an oversized tree. In an additional step this oversized tree will be optimized to the best size [91]. Aim of pruning is to find a tree with reduced complexity of the final classifier as well as better predictive accuracy. A sequence of trees is produced by use of cost-complexity-pruning [91]. Out of this sequence the best tree is chosen by evaluating the error rate considering the size of the FDT (sec. 3.8.3.1). The final tree for classification in a clinical context will be generated on the whole set of available classified date. The best tree then is chosen again after cross validation and finding the optimal tree by evaluating size and error rate.

8.3 Validation and Comparison

The standard way to evaluate a classificator is to perform a 10×10 cross validation. This means the data set is separated into 10 equal subsets. The tree is trained with 9 subsets and tested with the remaining "unknown" subset. The correct rate and error rate are computed and rated. This "training, testing and evaluation"-step is repeated until each of the 10 subsets was used to test the tree. This whole procedure is repeated 10 x which leads in total to 100 trees that are evaluated. This

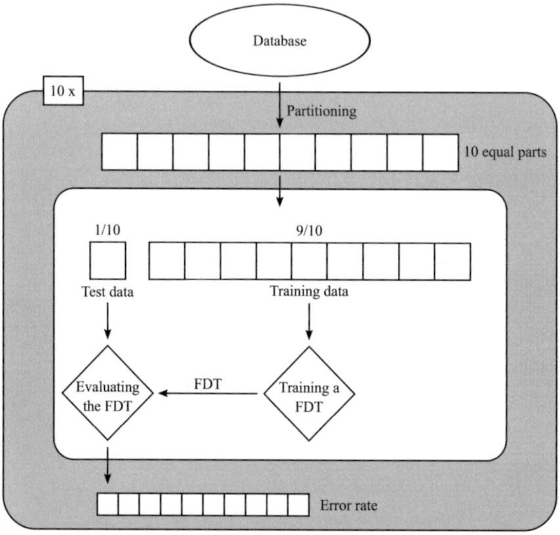

Fig. 8.3: Schematic depiction of the 10×10 cross validation.

evaluation has not only been done on the CFAE database but also on datasets from the UCI machine learning database (`archive.ics.uci.edu/ml/`). The UCI database is a regular database to test and evaluate machine learning algorithms. From this database 5 data sets have been chosen to evaluate the fuzzy decision tree. Data sets with continuous feature values and multi-class assignment have been chosen to be most similar to the CFAE data (tab. 8.1). Finally the results have been compared to different decision tree algorithms (CART [91], SLIQ [97], C4.5 [94], $FDT_{Chandra}$ [128]).

Table 8.1: Example data from the UCI machine learning database used for the evaluation of the fuzzy decision tree.

	Classes	Attributes	Objects	
Iris	3	4	150	species of lilies
Wine	3	13	178	types of wine
Wisconsin Breast Cancer	2	32	569	breast cancer diagnosis
Haberman's Survival	2	3	306	breast cancer mortality
Glas Identification	6	9	214	sorts of glas

8.4 Results of Evaluation

The fuzzy decision tree presented in the scope of this work was compared to results applied on commonly used test data sets of decision trees with sharp split values (CART, SLIQ, C4.5) and the fuzzy decision tree by Chandra et al. (FDT_X).
Table 8.2 gives an overview of the correct rates for each tree and each test data set. Presented is the error rate and its standard deviation for each classifier after a 10×10 cross validation. The results for FDT_X and SLIQ were obtained from [128] and the results for CART and C4.5 were obtained from [131]. The decision trees CART, SLIQ, and C4.5 have sharp split values, the fuzzy decision tree by Chandra et al. (FDT_X) uses a sigmoidal function as decision border. FDT is the tree presented in this work. For this tree, in addition to the error rate, the fuzzy zone width p for each data set is given. Compared with classical algorithms for decision trees and the fuzzy decision tree by Chandra et al. the correct rate results for the presented FDT are in the midrange for "Iris", "Wine", and "Wisconsin Breast Cancer" data sets. For these data sets the proposed FDT can compete. For the data sets "Haberman's survival" and "Glas Identification" the FDT gives the best results.
There are significantly lower correct rates for "Haberman's Survival" and "Glas Identification" data for all other classification algorithms. This can be caused by fuzzy features of these data sets. As the FDT is designed to work on fuzzy classification features it gives the best results. CFAE data is also "fuzzy data". This implies that FDT will work better for CFAE classification as compared to the other algorithms.

Table 8.2: Comparison of different decision tree algorithms. Shown are the error rate (%) ± the standard deviation (%) after 10 × 10 cross validation. CART and C4.5 data are obtained from [131], SLIQ and FDT_x are obtained from [128] (Wisconsin Breast Cancer (WBC), Haberman's Survival (HS), Glas Identification (GI)).

	CART	SLIQ	C4.5	FDT_x	FDT
Iris	93.5±0.8	98.0± 3.2	95.1±0.6	98.0± 3.2	96.1±4.8 (p=0.10)
Wine	89.3±0.8	88.3± 8.1	92.7±1.1	88.9± 4.5	89.1±7.2 (p=0.01)
WBC	-	93.3± 4.8	-	96.4± 4.9	92.4±3.6 (p=0.20)
HS	-	65.8±10.8	-	72.6± 7.8	74.4±7.2 (p=0.05)
GI	67.7±1.6	65.0±16.0	68.6±2.0	68.6±11.9	69.4±8.7 (p=0.10)

8.5 Results of CFAE Classification

The fuzzy decision tree is trained on the database described in section 4.3.1. For each electrogram the descriptors listed in table 8.3 are computed. The definitions for the descriptors can be found in chapter 7. With these descriptors and the given classification the training is realized. The evaluation is done by use of a 10 × 10 cross validation and computing the correct and error rates for each resulting tree.

8.5.1 Descriptor Results

The number and quality of descriptors used for a classification have a large effect on the classification result. Compared to other decision making tools, a decision tree is not as vulnerable for badly chosen descriptors. The tree will be smaller and the correct rate will be better, the better a single descriptor can distinguish between different classes. Such a single descriptor was not found. But, the separation of the four classes is also possible with a set of descriptors that can separate only two classes of CFAEs. As a consequence more than one descriptor is needed.
Some descriptors work better then others to distinguish between the different classes. Also, some descriptors are very similar and provide no new information. The fuzzy decision tree chooses the most efficient descriptors to separate the classes on its own depending on the best split values. Finding the most used descriptors and ignore the less used descriptors will improve computation time. Analyzing the number of most used descriptors finally resulted in a set of 18 descriptors. A histogram of the usage of these 18 descriptors at a decision node to divide the data is depicted in figure 8.4. This distribution is based on the results of a 10 × 10 cross validation.

Table 8.3 names all 35 originally used descriptors (F1 – F35). The reduced set of the 18 most frequently used descriptors is labeled with D1 – D18. The hereafter discussed results are based on the reduced descriptor set. A boxplot evaluation for all descriptors can be found in appendix A.1.

Table 8.3: Descriptors (F1 – F35) used to distinguish between CFAE classes and to train a FDT. The mostly used descriptors are additionally named with D1 – D18.

Descriptor		
F1	D1	Mean variance in time domain (mVarTD)
F2		Characteristic Frequency 1 by number of matches
F3		Characteristic Frequency 1 by power of maximum
F4		Characteristic Frequency 2 by number of matches
F5		Characteristic Frequency 2 by power of maximum
F6		Characteristic Frequency 3 number of matches
F7		Characteristic Frequency 3 by power of maximum
F8		Mean Characteristic Frequency
F9		Mean variance of Hilbert envelope
F10	D2	Histogramm excess (HistExc)
F11	D3	Phase space sample ratio region 1 (PSSR 1)
F12	D4	Phase space sample ratio region 2 (PSSR 2)
F13	D5	Phase space sample ratio region 3 (PSSR 3)
F14	D6	Phase space sample ratio region 4 (PSSR 4)
F15	D7	Entropy of phase space region 4 (EPS 4)
F16	D8	Mean cycle length of phase space region 4 (MCPS 4)
F17	D9	Similarity of AS (SimAS)
F18	D10	Activity ratio (AR)
F19	D11	Mean length of AS (MLAS)
F20	D12	Standard deviation of length of AS (sdMLAS)
F21	D13	Wavelet-based fractionation (WavFrac)
F22	D14	Number of AS (NoAS)
F23		Number of maxima in NLEO
F24		Number of maxima in low-pass filtered NLEO
F25		Sum of power spektrum
F26		Median value of 5 largest maxima
F27		Mean value of 5 largest maxima
F28		Variance of energy of AS
F29		Excess of length of inactive segments
F30		Standard deviation of excess of length of inactive segments
F31	D15	Mean of local maxima per AS (LocMaxAS)

Table 8.3: (continued)

Descriptor		
F32	D16	Mean zero crossings of AS (ZCAS)
F33	D17	Variance of local maxima per AS (varMaxAS)
F34	D18	Variance of zero crossings of AS (varZCAS)
F35		Entropy of EGM

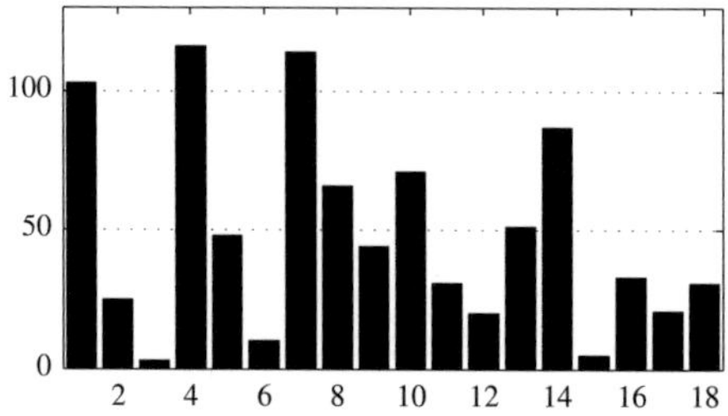

Fig. 8.4: Histogram of most frequently used descriptors for all 100 trees resulting from 10 × 10 cross validation.

The results for descriptors D1 – D18 are shown in table 8.4. For each CFAE class the median ($\tilde{\mu}$) and the interquartile range (IQR) per descriptor are listed. The median and the IQR give an overview of the distribution of the descriptor values and the power to separate CFAE classes of each descriptor. Generally, there is no descriptor that can separate between all four CFAE classes alone. However, the descriptors can separate between different CFAE class groups. For example the descriptors D5 (PSSR 3), D10 (AR), D1 (mVarTD), D4 (PSSR 2), and D18 (varZCAS) can separate C0 from C3. D14 (NoAS) can be used to separate C0 and C3 from C1 and C2. The boxplots of the descriptors used by the tree, shown in figure 8.6, are depicted in figure 8.5. It can be seen, that the mean and the IQR are different for each CFAE class for each descriptor. In addition also the PDF is changing significantly. So, the chosen descriptors reflect the difference of the diverging signals.

The different CFAE classes can be separated by the PSSR descriptors. Data values for very regular signals (e.g. SR) consists mostly of zeros and only a few deflections that are non-zero, whereas continuous activity has mainly small values

Table 8.4: Results of the mostly used descriptors. Median $\tilde{\mu}$ and interquartile range (IQR) per CFAE class are given.

	CFAE class							
Descriptor	C0		C1		C2		C3	
D1	0.17	(0.01)	0.18	(0.02)	0.21	(0.02)	0.23	(0.03)
D2	22.62	(10.36)	12.88	(5.33)	9.76	(3.17)	6.83	(2.48)
D3	0.88	(0.08)	0.70	(0.14)	0.52	(0.11)	0.35	(0.12)
D4	0.02	(0.03)	0.07	(0.03)	0.13	(0.03)	0.14	(0.03)
D5	0.01	(0.01)	0.04	(0.02)	0.08	(0.02)	0.11	(0.02)
D6	0.10	(0.03)	0.18	(0.09)	0.26	(0.08)	0.40	(0.13)
D7	1.60	(0.19)	2.09	(0.44)	2.51	(0.26)	2.67	(0.08)
D8	5.71	(0.32)	5.14	(0.31)	4.74	(0.20)	4.59	(0.14)
D9	−0.17	(0.42)	−0.68	(0.26)	−0.97	(0.17)	−1.17	(0.21)
D10	0.18	(0.06)	0.32	(0.15)	0.56	(0.17)	0.82	(0.14)
D11 (ms)	54.46	(13.42)	75.67	(31.97)	132.09	(62.60)	312.88	(271.54)
D12 (ms)	4.45	(13.95)	18.01	(13.58)	86.25	(78.23)	345.59	(334.66)
D13	345.00	(112.00)	630.00	(273.50)	809.00	(265.00)	1152.00	(433.00)
D14	18.00	(5.00)	26.00	(5.00)	24.00	(4.00)	15.00	(9.25)
D15	1.68	(0.29)	2.02	(0.41)	2.52	(0.40)	3.29	(0.78)
D16	1.44	(0.34)	1.76	(0.42)	2.27	(0.41)	3.06	(0.76)
D17	0.18	(1.76)	1.48	(1.01)	4.21	(1.69)	6.54	(2.03)
D18	−0.13	(1.78)	1.40	(1.01)	3.68	(1.70)	6.07	(2.09)

scattering around zero and nearly no zero values. Thus, CFAEs will be found primarily in the outer phase space regions and SR signals primarily in phase space region 1. The median values for D4 (PSSR 2) and D5 (PSSR 3) are significantly different on a 5% level (boxplot notches) for all four CFAE classes. Also there is no overlapping of the interquartile range. The entropy of the number of hits in the different regions of the phase space (EPS) reflects also the behavior of these signals in the phase space. D7 (EPS 4) can be used to distinguish nearly between all CFAE classes. Medians are significantly different for all classes and IQR are not overlapping for C0, C2, and C3. The same applies to D10 (AR). Medians are significantly different and IQR are not overlapping for all classes. This was expected: the more activity in an electrogram, the more active segments will be found and the larger the value of AR will be. Instead for very regular EGMs the active segments will take only a small account and, therefore, the AR will tend to have small values. D14 (NoAS) can separate signals with small number of AS and those that have a large number of AS. The heart rate of AFlut is in the range of 3 – 6 beats per second. With a 5 second electrogram this rate is in the range 15 – 30 beats per 5 s. Continuous activity instead can have also smaller number of active segments, but segments will be longer. The number of active segments is the largest for fast, regular activity (C1, C2). The descriptor D14 (NoAS) can separate C0 and C3 from C1 and C2. There is an overlap of the IQR of C1 and C2, but, although the value range is very similar the medians are significantly different. D1 (mVarTD) can also distinguish between the classes. The distributions of this descriptor is overlapping for the classes, but the medians are significantly different and IQR is not overlapping. Regular signals have mainly symmetrically and gaussian-like NLEO signal curves per AS. This is reflected by a small variance. NLEO of AS of more complex and high fractionated electrograms will have more variation and thus, larger variance. Finally, same statements hold true, for D18 (varZCAS), where the zero crossing of AS are evaluated. AS of high fractionated electrograms have a lot more deflections and, thus, more zero crossings will be detected compared to more regular electrograms. For all delineated descriptors the medians are significantly different on a 5 % level for all CFAE classes.

8.5.2 Classification Results

The evaluation by the cross validation process gives an estimation for the correct rate for the tested method. This value is correct whilst the training data reflect reality data. To generate a fuzzy decision tree to work on new data or in a clinical environment, the tree will be trained with all available data [132]. The correct rate for this newly built classificator can be estimated from the mean correct rate resulting from cross validation. Applying a 10×10 cross validation on the presented fuzzy decision tree algorithm with a fuzzy zone width of 20% results in a mean correct rate of $80.65\% \pm 3.3\%$. So, a mean correct rate of 80% can be expected, but there can also be trees with better correct rates. Correct rates for the different CFAE classes are C0: $83.1\% \pm 4.4$, C1: $81.0\% \pm 8.1$, C2: $75.8\% \pm 8.4$, C3: $82.7\% \pm 17.8$. The distribution of the wrong assignments of signals per class is shown in table 8.5. Wrong assigned signals were mostly assigned to neighboring classes. This is less critical as the physicians themselves sometimes were hesitating while classifying CFAEs. So, there is still an ambiguity left in the training data.

Choosing one tree out of the sequence of cross validated trees with a fuzzy width of 20% results in a tree with a correct rate of 86.1% (C0: 92.9%, C1: 83.3%, C2:

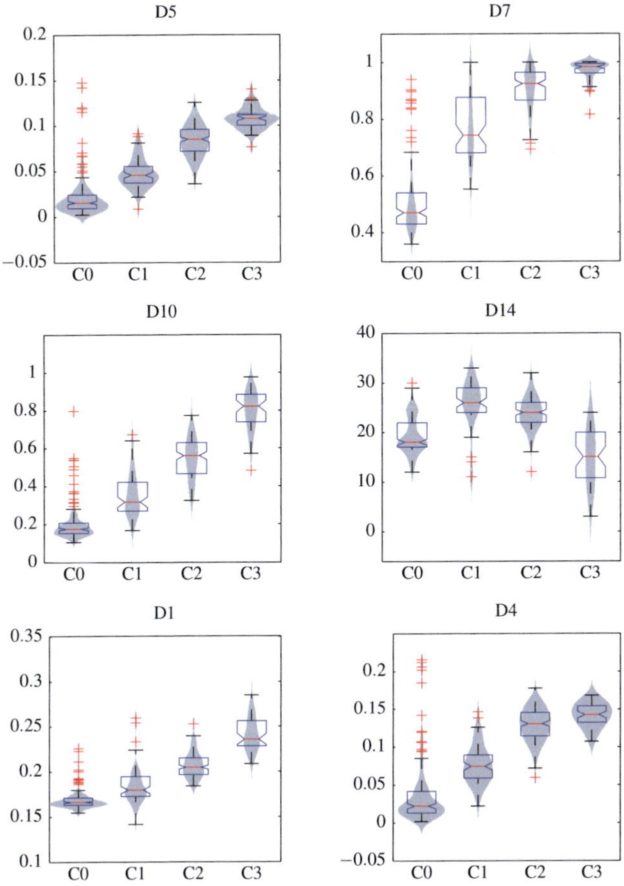

Fig. 8.5: Boxplots of descriptors used by the tree with best correct rate (continued on next page).

69.3%, C3: 100%). This tree is depicted in Fig. 8.6. At each node the chosen descriptor and its split value is depicted and for each leaf node the class membership results are shown. This tree uses only 7 different descriptors.

In addition to the classification result there is also a certainty for the classification given. So, the physician can decide whether the given classification is trustful or

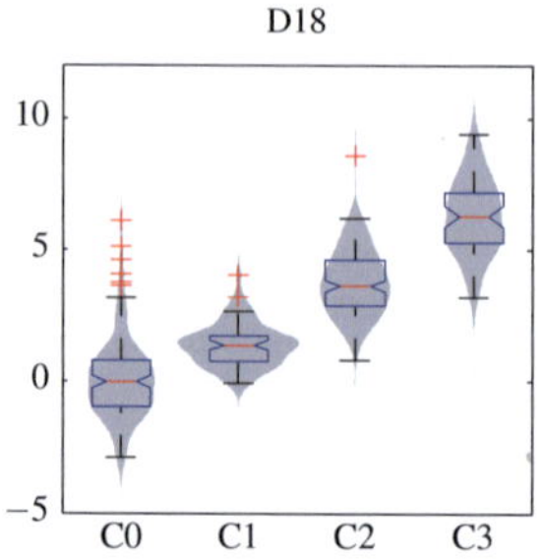

Fig. 8.5: (continued)

Table 8.5: Wrong assignments per CFAE class.

	wrong assigned to			
	class C0	class C1	class C2	class C3
C0	X	72%	24%	4%
C1	36%	X	63%	1%
C2	2%	49%	X	49%
C3	0%	0%	100%	X

not. This can support an electrophysiologist while ablating to decide whether a signal is worth analyzing or not.

The performance of the fuzzy decision tree is better the more data is used to train the tree. Starting with 605 signals, 429 signals have been classified coinciding by two physicians. The smallest group of CFAE classes is C3 with 53 signals. Therefore, to get objective results by a 10×10 cross validation, all classes have to have the same size. Otherwise one class would be overrepresented. As a consequence the 10×10 cross validation is done with 212 signals, 53 for each CFAE class. Splitting the data in 10 equally sized groups results in 48 signals per class to train the tree and only 5 signals per class to test it. With only 5 signals per CFAE class to test, the results are not statistically significant. To overcome this problem the 10×10 cross validation results in 100 trees that are evaluated. Nevertheless, the results are vulnerable for outliers. The more signals are used for training the less signals remain for testing. A 10×5 cross validation will give 42 signals per class to train the tree and 11 signals to test it. This might be a better choice, but the 10×10 cross validation is a standard procedure and should be used also for com-

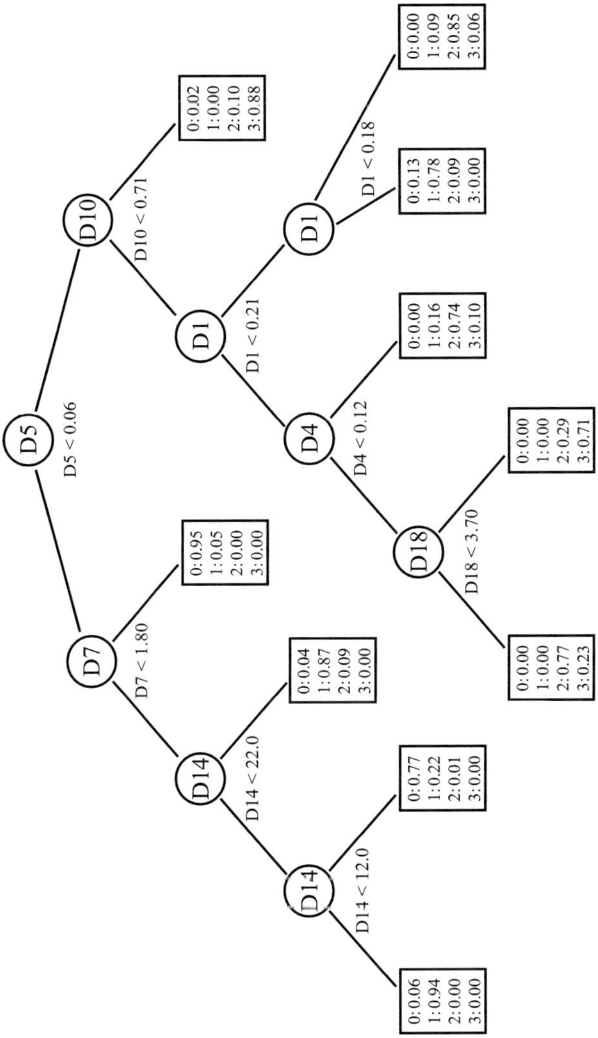

Fig. 8.6: Fuzzy decision tree with the smallest error rate resulting from a 10×10 cross validation. For each leaf node the probable class membership results are given.

parability of the results. Also, Breiman et. al showed, that 10×10 cross validation results in trustful results even with small parts of test data [91].
Concluding, one can state, that the FDT presented here can support electrophysiologists while ablating AF and can help to simplify and to objectify signal analysis of CFAEs. Since a certainty of classification is given, the physician can evaluate the reliability of the given result. As the definition of CFAEs is not the golden truth, each physician has his/her own interpretation and understanding what a CFAE is and looks like. So, this algorithm can help to find a valid and absolute mathematical definition of CFAE.

9

Contact vs. Non-contact Electrograms

Sufficient contact between a catheter and the endocardium is crucial for reliable recording and analysis of myocardial electrograms. Furthermore, to achieve transmural lesions in the endocardial wall during catheter ablation the ablating electrode must touch the endocardium. With only a small gap between the tip of the catheter and the endocardium the transition resistance of the ablation current is increasing enormously. This holds true for atrial as well as ventricular EP examinations [133, 134].

To control the catheter contact, the physician is sensing the tactile blow back from the catheter and is additionally monitoring changes in the signal. When loosing endocardial contact, physicians observed that the signal and its morphology are changing [135, 136]. Fluoroscopic images and the 3D visualization provided by mapping systems give only a rough impression of the catheter's contact. Additionally, the regularly measured endocardial impedance can be used to analyze the endocardium contact. Values between $150-250\,\Omega$ have been figured out as threshold [137, 138]. Nevertheless, the impedance can only give a tendency as the absolute values are not known and the impedance values vary significantly between different patients and even in one patient at different locations within the heart.

Figure 9.1 depicts atrial signals measured with and without catheter contact at different locations. The signals were measured in the left and right atrium. The upper signals were measured at the posterior wall, the lower ones in close proximity to the septum, and the signals in the middle result from a location at the terminal crest. The left column shows signals with endocardial contact and the right column shows signals without or less endocardial contact. Obviously, the signal's shape is changing when loosing endocardial contact. The amplitude is decreasing and the spikes are getting smoother and more dulled.

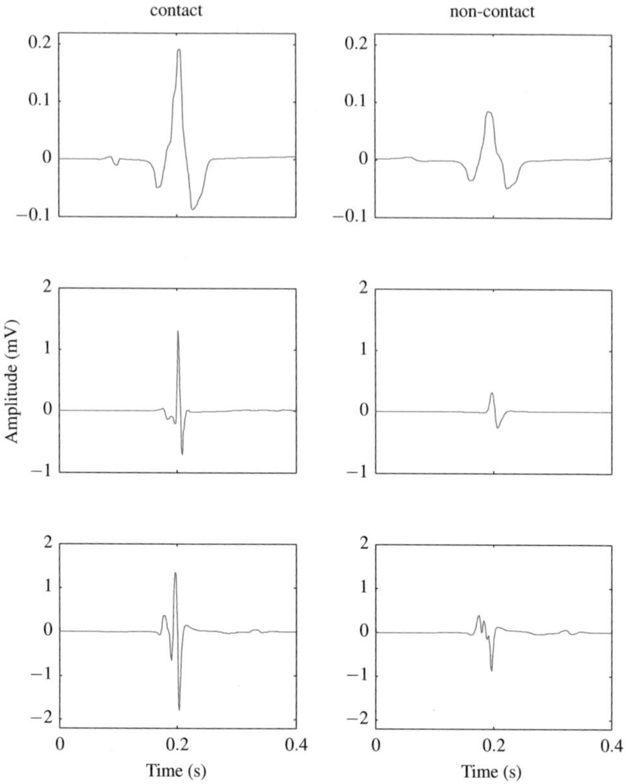

Fig. 9.1: Measured signals with catheter contact to the endocardium and measured at the same location without contact. Each row depicts signals from the same location within the left atrium.

Rango et al. also described the influence of endocardial contact on the catheter signal [126]. They described blunt signals with loose contact to the endocardium due to missing high frequency parts within the signal. Compared to this, contact signals gave sharp, peaky signals. It would be helpful to distinguish between contact and non-contact signals by automatically analyzing the signal. Using the descriptors introduced in chapter 7 and a classified database of contact and non-contact EGMs, a classifier was trained. To support the observations of the physicians and the findings of the descriptors, a simulation of atrial electrograms and varying catheter distances and orientations was performed.

9.1 Simulation of Intracardiac Electrograms

Besides the analysis of measured signals, the influence of catheter contact as well as the catheter orientation on a bipolar electrogram will be analyzed in a simulation setting. This could confirm the clinical observations and could lead to a better understanding of the formation of the bipolar EGM. Therefore, a computer model of atrial tissue and the catheter is defined and the excitation propagation on this model is computed. Varying the catheter distance to the endocardium and the orientation of the catheter will lead to different EGMs, that can be compared to measured signals.
The excitation simulation in an atrial tissue is calculated with acCELLerate. This software package was developed at the Institute of Biomedical Engineering for the computation of reaction-diffusion-systems. It uses the bidomain equations (sec. 2.6) to compute the intracellular and extracellular currents and voltages of cardiac cells and tissue.

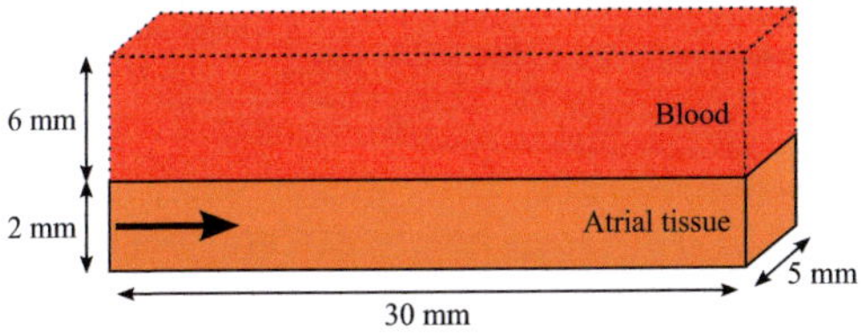

Fig. 9.2: Schematic representation of the tissue model. The atrial tissue will be excited from the left side. The upper layer is filled with blood in which the catheter will be added.

Fig. 9.3: Excitation propagation computed in the tissue model with acCELLerate. Depicted is the x-y-plane and the color coded transmembrane voltage at one time instant. Yellow color indicates 0 mV, blue color −80 mV.

Instead of simulating on a whole atrium a tissue patch of $300 \times 50 \times 80$ voxel with a resolution of 0,1 mm is chosen. On this tissue patch the excitation is computed. This simplification is justified as only a small region around the tip of the catheter influences the measurement of the catheter. The resulting patch is $30 \times 5 \times 8$ mm and is filled in z-direction with 2 mm of atrial tissue and 6 mm of blood (fig. 9.2). The simulation of an atrial excitation is started with an initial stimulation at the left side of the tissue patch (fig. 9.3). As consequence the excitation spreads over the whole tissue patch and extracellular potentials can be computed [139].

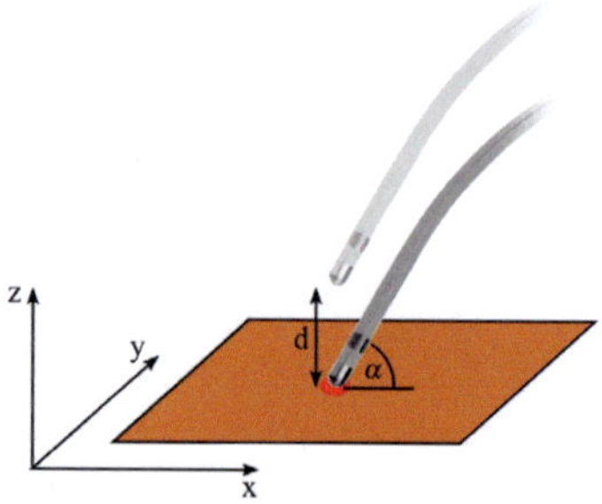

Fig. 9.4: Catheter orientation for different simulation outcomes. The distance d between the tip of the catheter and the endocardium, the angle α between the catheter and the x-y-plane, and the angle β between the catheter and the x-z-plane will be varied.

The excitation is computed based on the Courtemanche-Ramirez-Nattel cell model (sec. 2.5.2). This model generates an AP based on the general setup. As the EGMs measured in the atria can be very different according to where they have been measured, the CRN model can not reproduce this variety. Nevertheless, this model can be used to analyze the influence of catheter distance and orientation on the bipolar EGM in general.

To measure the simulated signals a catheter with electrodes is modelled. In a first approach the electrodes are modelled as point-sensors with a distance of 2 mm. The catheter signal is obtained from the difference of the potentials in these sensors. In a further approach the catheter is modelled like a regular ablation catheter. Therefore, the catheter shaft is modelled and ring electrodes are added (fig 9.4). The catheter has a diameter of 1 mm. The electrodes have a length of 1 mm with an inter-electrode spacing of 2 mm. They are assigned to the material class of metal. Thus, the extracellular conductivity within an electrode is very high and the sin-

gle electrode signal is gained as mean from the “point-electrodes” lying within the catheter. The atrial EGM then is calculated from the difference of the single electrode signals.
With this setting the catheter distance to the endocardium is modelled. Starting with a distance of 0 mm (contact signal), the distance is increased in 0.1 mm steps up to 2 mm. Also the angles between the catheter and the x-y-plane (α) and the catheter and the x-z-plane (β) are varied (tab. 9.1).

Table 9.1: Different orientations of the simulated catheter to the endocard. α is the angle in direction of the excitation propagation, β is perpendicular to the excitation propagation.

Position	α	β
1	0°	0°
2	45°	0°
3	0°	45°
4	45°	45°
5	90°	0°

9.2 Detecting Signals with Endocardium Contact

For the signal analysis as well as for the ablation process during an EP study it is crucial to have catheter contact to the endocardium. Based on the experience of the Karlsruhe physicians a database of contact and non-contact signals was generated as described in section 4.3.3. Based on the this data a set of discriptors that delineate features of contact and non-contact signals was developed. With these descriptors and the classified database then a CART decision tree is build (sec. 3.8).

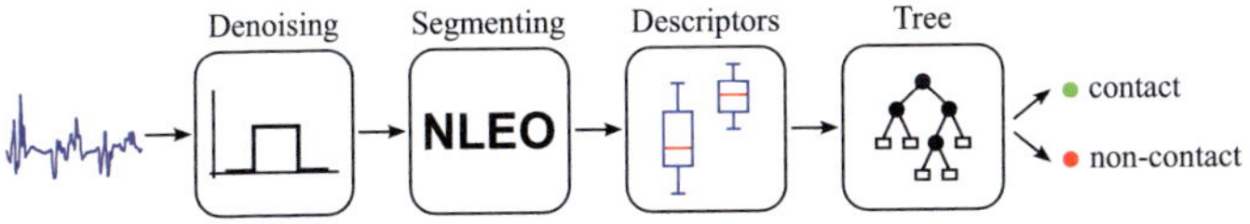

Fig. 9.5: Block diagram to detect catheter contact on the endocardium.

Figure 9.5 depicts a block diagram of the general algorithm to detect signals with endocardium contact. The signals are preprocessed as described in section 4.3.3.

Afterwards the signals are segmented with help of the NLEO segmenting algorithm to find active segments within the signal. On the active segments then the different descriptors are calculated. Table 9.2 gives an overview of the utilized descriptors. The calculation of these descriptors is introduced in chapter 7. With the methods described in section 3.8 a decision tree as classifier is build, that decides whether a signal had endocardium contact or not. The resulting decision tree is evaluated with a 10×10 cross validation. Finally, the decision tree is cross checked with signals resulting from the simulations described in the preceding section.

9.3 Results of Analyzing the Endocardium Contact of Catheter

9.3.1 Simulated EGMs Results

From the simulations it turned out that the catheter orientation influences the signal morphology. As the results are nearly the same for all orientations, exemplarily the signals for only one catheter orientation are depicted here. The signals for the remaining catheter orientations can be found in appendix B.
In section 9.1 two methods have been introduced to simulate a catheter. One possibility was to have only point-sensors, and the second option was to model a more realistic catheter that averages several point-sensors. The signals have small differences in morphology and amplitude. As the simulation was made in a simplified environment, these differences can be considered negligible.

Influence of Distance

The results of simulating electrograms calculated with different distances to the endocardium are discussed with catheter position 2 and a modeled catheter. The simulation was realized with distances between the catheter and the endocardium in 0.1 mm steps, starting at 0 mm and ending at 2 mm. The results will be discussed for distances of 0 mm, 0.1 mm, 0.5 mm, 1 mm, and 2 mm, as the changes from one distance step to the next were small. For the distances of 0 mm and 0.1 mm contact is assumed, for the remaining distances non-contact. A distance of 0 mm represents strong catheter contact, whereas a distance of 0.1 mm represents weak catheter contact. The results of the simulated electrograms can be seen in fig. 9.6. The single electrograms for each catheter position are depicted for a detailed view and additionally a plot with the signals superimposed for better comparison. It can

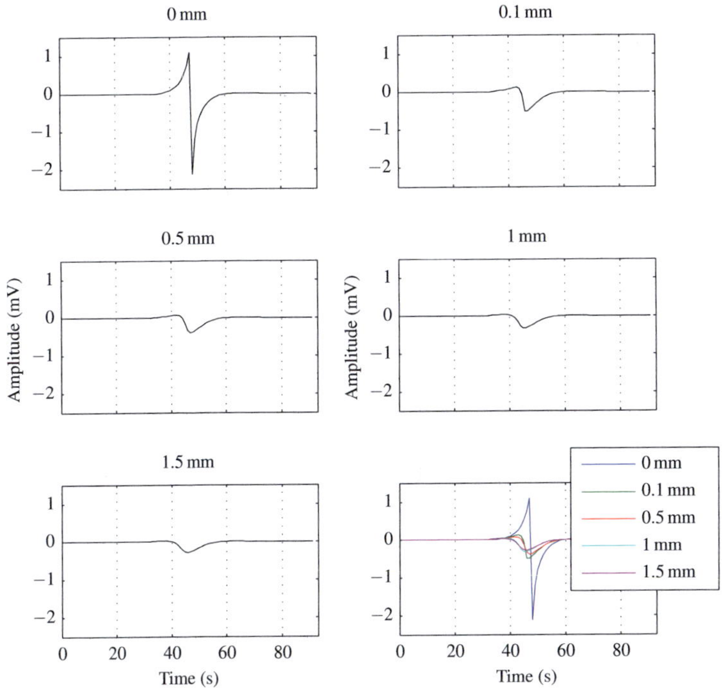

Fig. 9.6: Simulated electrograms with different distances between the catheter and the endocardium.

be seen, that the simulated signals behave according to the observations made in the EP lab. With increasing distance from the catheter to the endocardium, signal's amplitude is getting smaller and the peakedness is vanishing. This effect was observed for all different orientations of the catheter.

Influence of Catheter Orientation

When comparing the different orientations of the catheter, it becomes clear, that there is an obvious influence. Both, the amplitude and the signal morphology are changing according to the orientation of the catheter. For position 1 and 3, both electrodes of the catheter have contact to the endocardium ($\alpha = 0$), whereas for the other three positions only the tip electrode touches the endocardium ($\alpha \neq 0$). When

varying the angle between the catheter and the excitation direction (α) mainly the amplitude height and the signal width is influenced. This can be seen when comparing position 1 and 3 or position 2 and 4. The signal complex is getting smaller, as the excitation hits the second electrode earlier. Changing α leads to slightly changing morphology. Changing β leads to heavy changes in the signal's morphology. This is mainly caused by an increasing distance of the second electrode to the endocardium and leads to a signal loss in the same electrodes. This effect can be seen when comparing position 1 and 2 or position 3 and 4.
So, one can state, that there is a large influence of the catheter orientation. Changing β effects the electrogram more than changing the angle to the excitation direction (α). This covers the experience physicians made in the EP lab.

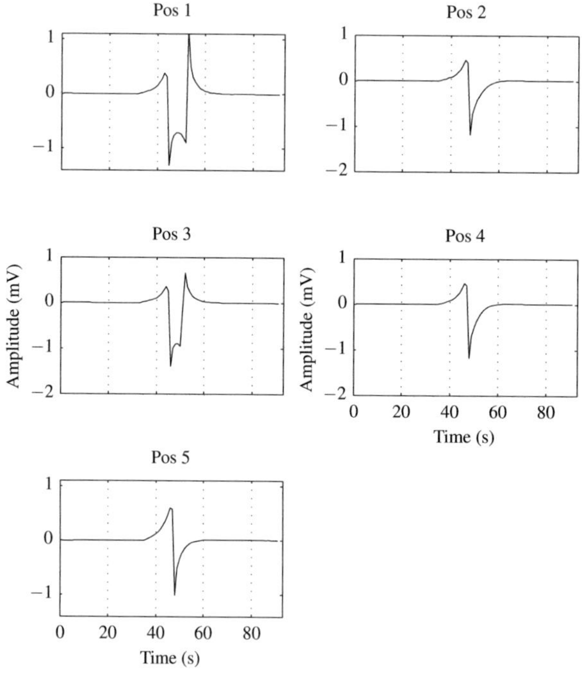

Fig. 9.7: Simulated electrograms with different orientations between the catheter and the endocardium.

Influence of Filtering

As there is no opportunity to do a quantitativ measure on the correctness of the simulation, a qualitative comparison is discussed. Measured signals in the EP lab are regularly tainted with artifacts and are denoised with low-pass and high-pass filters. Commonly the signals are filtered with a 30 Hz high-pass and a 150 Hz low-pass filter. This filtering has a large influence on the EGM's morphology [135]. Figure 9.8 depicts an EGM before and after applying filtering.
As the simulated signals are pure and unfiltered, the same filtering is applied on them. If they reflect at least to a small extent the features of realistic signals, they should behave in a similar manner to the filtering. The filters are applied on a simulated EGM that looks similar to the unfiltered EGM depicted in figure 9.8. The resulting EGM is shown in figure 9.9. It is obvious that the filtering affects the simulated EGM analogically. The resulting EGM is very similar in shape to the one depicted in figure 9.8.

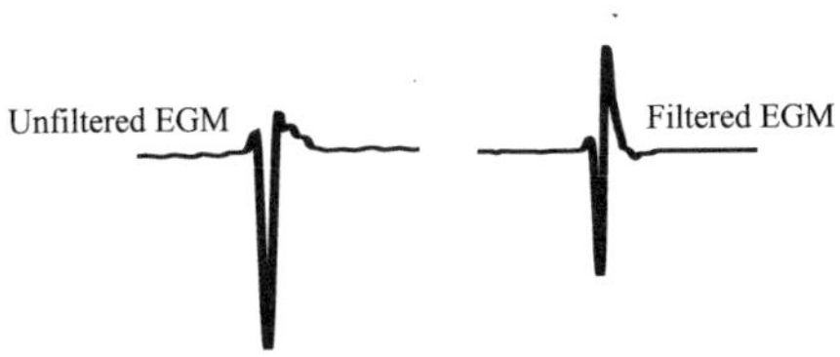

Fig. 9.8: Effect of applying a band-pass filter (30 – 150 Hz) on electrograms (adapted from [135]).

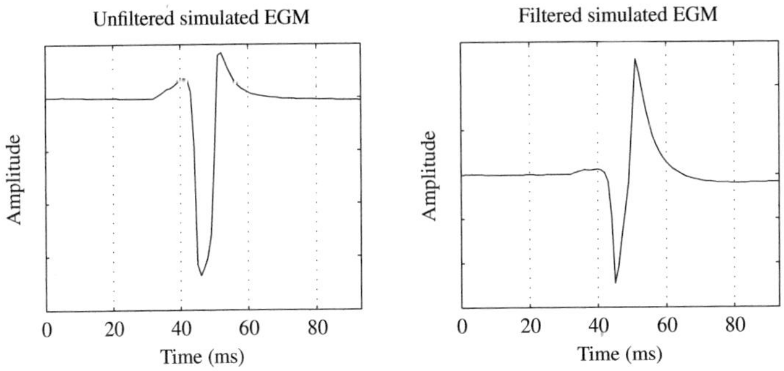

Fig. 9.9: Effect of applying a band-pass filter (30 – 150 Hz) on simulated electrograms.

Although the simulation environment is very simplified, the signals achieved from the simulation cover the experience and knowledge gained from EGMs measured in the EP lab [135, 136]. Conclusive, this method can be used to easily investigate and show complex events in the interaction of atrial tissue and catheters.

9.3.2 Decision Tree Results

Descriptor Results

To distinguish between contact and non-contact signals, a database and a set of descriptors is needed. All descriptors used to train a decision tree are shown in table 9.2. Also the median $\tilde{\mu}$ and the interquartile range (IQR) for each descriptor calculated on the classified database (sec. 4.3.3) are given. The median and the IQR give an overview of the distribution of the descriptor values and the power to separate between contact and non-contact classes of each descriptor. Additionally, the boxplot representation for the descriptors used by the tree with smallest error rate (fig. 9.11) are presented. The boxplot for all other descriptors can be found in appendix A.2.
Resulting from the observation that signals are loosing peakedness with increasing catheter distance, analyzing the frequency domain lead to good separation results. Loosing peakedness is represented by vanishing high frequency parts in the power spectrum. This is reflected by the descriptors D_c16 (max. energy peak > 100 Hz) and D_c12 (percental frequency distribution $130-300$ Hz). The mean and the IQR are significantly different for contact and non-contact signals. All descriptors based on the frequency domain analysis could differentiate between the two classes (e.g. D_c19-D_c22). Using, for example, only D_c1 with a fixed threshold to separate the classes, would lead to a correct rate of 90.2%. Thus, the vanishing high frequency componentes are supposed to be the main difference between the classes.
Descriptors analyzing the amplitude and morphology of the signals also lead to significant different representations (e.g. D_c3-D_c6) of the two classes. The PCA-based decision also lead to good separation results. For contact signals with a sharp peak, most data values are zero and only a few are non-zero. Data values for non-contact signals are more scattered around zero in the amplitude histogram. This can be reflected by higher order statistics (D_c3-D_c6), but also with phase space representation (D_c7-D_c11). This behavior can be seen by the boxplot representa-

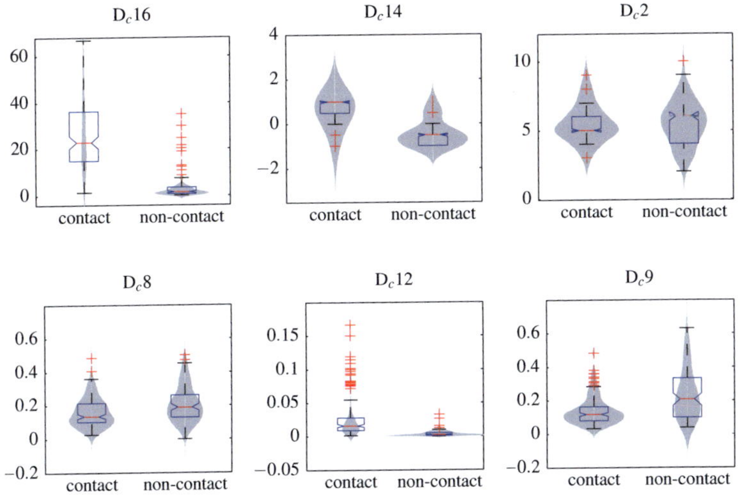

Fig. 9.10: Boxplots of descriptors used by the tree with best correct rate.

tion in figure 9.10. Descriptors D_c8 and D_c9 show a significant difference in the median and also the PDF estimation is changing distinctively.

Most descriptors work well to separate the two classes. The outcome of the frequency domain descriptors have to be highlighted, as e.g. D_c1 can be used solitary to achieve a correct rate from more than 90%. To improve correct rates additional descriptors will be used. This has also the advantage to use non-dependent descriptors and to justice the variety of electrograms. Thus, the presented set of descriptors will be used to train and validate a decision tree.

Table 9.2: Results of descriptors used to classify contact and non-contact signals. Median $\tilde{\mu}$ and interquartile range (IQR) are given.

Descriptor		contact signal		non-contact signal	
D_c1	Percental frequency distribution 0 – 90 Hz	0.74	(0.12)	0.91	(0,08)
D_c2	Zero crossings, wavelet-based	5.00	(1.00)	6.00	(2.00)
D_c3	Expectation value of amplitude histogram	28.94	(11.31)	30.14	(6.38)
D_c4	Variance of amplitude histogram	65.95	(21.00)	126.10	(70.44)
D_c5	Skewness of amplitude histogram	−0.93	(2.69)	−0.86	(1.17)

Table 9.2: (continued)

Descriptor		contact signal		non-contact signal	
D_c6	Excess of amplitude histogram	6.71	(5.52)	1.53	(2.85)
D_c7	Phase space sample ratio region 1 (PSSR 1)	0.59	(0.17)	0.29	(0.39)
D_c8	Phase space sample ratio region 2 (PSSR 2)	0.13	(0.11)	0.19	(0.13)
D_c9	Phase space sample ratio region 3 (PSSR 3)	0.12	(0.08)	0.21	(0.23)
D_c10	Phase space sample ratio region 4 (PSSR 4)	0.13	(0.08)	0.24	(0.14)
D_c11	Entropy of phase space region 4 (EPS 4)	0.56	(0.23)	0.81	(0.24)
D_c12	Percental frequency distribution 130 – 300 Hz	0.02	(0.02)	0.00	(0.00)
D_c13	Entropy signal	3.20	(0.98)	2.86	(0.87)
D_c14	PCA-based decision	1.00	(0.50)	−0.50	(0.50)
D_c15	NLEO energy	1.26	(6.43)	0.00	(0.05)
D_c16	Max. energy peak > 100 Hz	22.77	(21.40)	1.57	(2.66)
D_c17	Correlation PCA with non-contact signals	0.63	(0.47)	0.80	(0.24)
D_c18	Correlation PCA with contact signals	0.84	(0.22)	0.58	(0.37)
D_c19	Expectation value spectrums's envelope	61.39	(21.34)	44.60	(12.18)
D_c20	Variance spectrums's envelope	855.47	(366.59)	577.84	(378.8)
D_c21	Skewness spectrums's envelope	1.19	(0.95)	1.73	(0.55)
D_c22	Excess spectrums's envelope	1.99	(3.34)	4.38	(3.44)

Classification Results

To classify contact and non-contact signals a classical CART decision tree is built as described in section 3.8. The tree is build and trained with the database of classified signals introduced in section 4.3.3. The evaluation of the decision tree is made by a 10×10 cross validation. Figure 9.11 depicts the decision tree resulting from a 10×10 cross validation with the smallest error rate. This tree has a correct rate of 97.2%.

The tree has also been tested with simulated electrograms. A database of signals is generated as test database. Therefore, signals are simulated in different distances to the endocardium. Signals resulting from a distance of 0 mm or 0.1 mm are considered to be contact signals, all other signals are considered to be non-contact signals. All together 38 signals are generated, 18 contact signals and 20 non-contact signals. These signals have been applied to the tree trained with measured and classified data. The correct rate was 94,7%. Only two simulated signals have been misclassified. The proposed method to classify contact and non-contact EGMs works

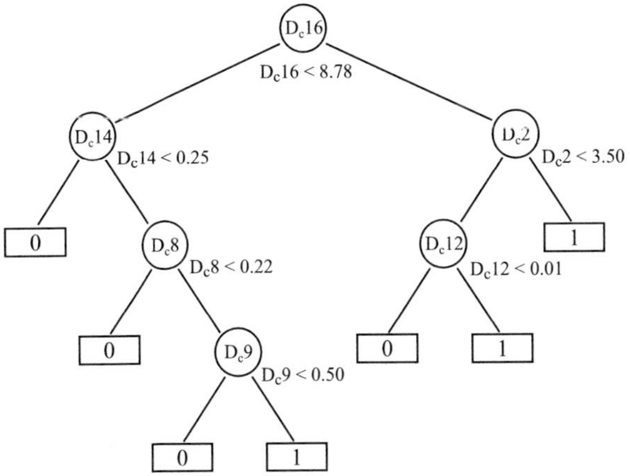

Fig. 9.11: Decision tree to detect catheter contact on the endocardium with the best correct rate resulting from cross validation. A '0' at a leaf node indicates no catheter contact, a '1' indicates catheter contact.

well on the database of 256 signals. These signals have been recorded in patients suffering from atrial flutter, atrial fibrillation and Wolff-Parkinson-White syndrom. Only signals with very regular shape have been chosen. This method might fail when trying to classify more complex AF signals. Even in SR or AFlut the possible signal morphology can vary heavily and e.g. non-contact signals recorded at the christa terminalis may look like contact signals recorded at the septum. To improve the reliability of the decision tree, the database should be extended. Otherwise, this method is an improvement to state-of-the-art analysis of catheter contact and might lead to better ablation results.

10

3D Visualization

During AF ablation a common way to reduce radiation exposure is to use mapping systems (sec. 2.4.2). With these systems catheters within the heart can be localized and the position of the electrodes can be tracked. While sliding the catheter over the endocard, a pointcloud will be produced which represents the atrial geometry. From this pointcloud the surface of the patient specific atria is reconstructed by the mapping systems. After triangulation the system displays the atria as a mesh or solid surface. In addition to this atria visualization, the current position of the catheter can be displayed in relation to the atria surface. As commercial software systems like EnSite NavX™ or CARTO only allow to export data and not to play new gained data or information back into the system, all signal processing and analysis must be done offline in an external environment. In this work all signal processing and visualization is done within the matlab environment.

10.1 Visualization of Atrial Geometry

The exported triangulated atria consist of two matrices. The first matrix represents the vertices of the triangulation and consists of (x,y,z)-coordinates. The second matrix holds the information in which order the vertices have to be connected to build the surface. To visualize the atria in the matlab environment each coordinate is plotted and the coordinates are connected according to the given order in the second matrix. On the left hand side in figure 10.1 the triangulation of the exported patient specific atria is represented. Based on this surface representation the atria can be colored (fig. 10.1, right hand side).

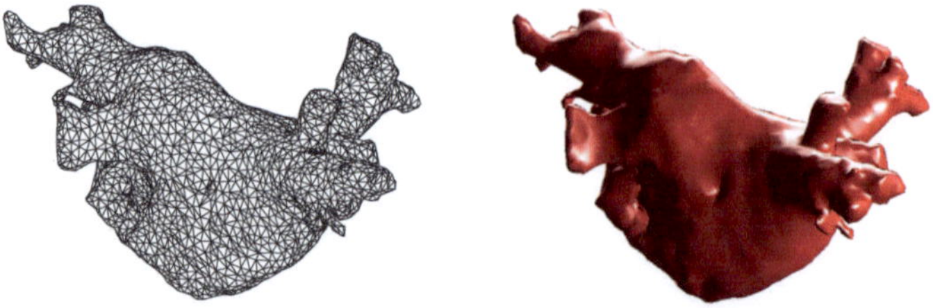

Fig. 10.1: EnSite NavX™ anatomical map of the left atrium. The triangulated representation of a patient specific anatomy (left) recorded during an EP examination and its colored surface (right).

10.2 Spatial Analysis — Visualization of Descriptors

During an electrophysiological examination all signals are stored together with the (x,y,z)-coordinates of the signal's measurement location. With this information the complete electrophysiological examination can be replayed and additional information gained from the signal's analysis can be displayed at the specific measurement location onto the atrium's surface. To add newly gained information (descriptors) on the patient specific atria, the new information is visualized on the anatomical map. The measurement coordinates of the catheter electrodes are in general not identical with the anatomical vertices. As matlab can only color triangulations starting from a vertex, for each measurement point the nearest vertex must be found. This is done by calculating the euclidean distance and searching the smallest distance between the measurement point and a vertex. Next the information (descriptor) gained on the measurement point is projected onto the nearest vertex. The error that is made by transposing the real measurement point to the nearest anatomical vertex is smaller than one edge length of a triangle. Analyzing the mean edge length of 27 patient specific atrial geometries lead to a mean value of 1.8 ± 4.5 mm. Thus, the error is smaller than 2 mm, what is also the system's spatial resolution [140]. So, this error is negligible.
To get a spatial impression of the descriptor distribution on the atria not only the measurement vertex v_x must be colored but also some neighboring vertices. The neighboring vertices will be assigned with a weighted descriptor value of v_x. This weighting is done to get a smooth value distribution and to emphasize the measurement vertex. Starting with v_x the vertices that can be reached within two traverses will be assigned with a value according to the descriptor value $f(v_x)$ at v_x. The first

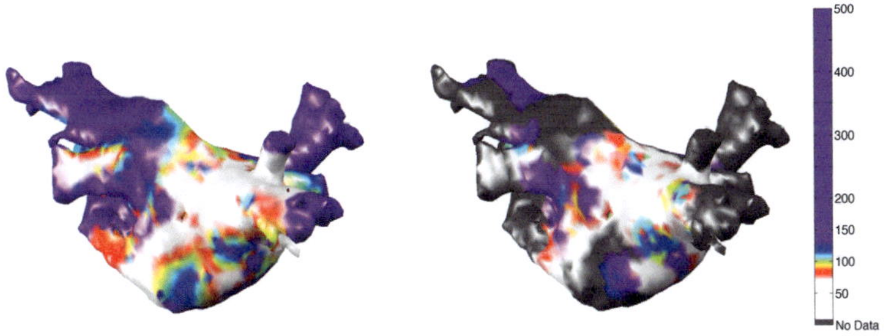

Fig. 10.2: A colored visualization of the CFAEmean descriptor on a left atrium as displayed by EnSite NavX™ system (left) and the visualization method presented in this work (right). The method introduced here displays only colors at small areas around measurement points, whereas the EnSite NavX™ algorithm interpolates color generously. Grey areas are areas with no measurement values.

generation of neighboring vertices (direct neighboring vertices) will be assigned with $0.95 \cdot f(\mathrm{v}_x)$, the second generation of vertices wil be assigned with $0.9 \cdot f(\mathrm{v}_x)$. If one of these vertices has itself a descriptor value or has an assignment from a neighboring vertex, the mean of these values will be assigned to this vertex.

With the medical assumption that the atrial condition during arrhythmias is steady in a 15 min segment [141], the descriptors gained from step-by-step measured signals can be visualized as spatial information on the atria. This is done also by EnSite NavX™ or CARTO systems. They both provide methods to display for example the fractionation of the electrograms on the atria or the local activation time. Figure 10.2 depicts on the left hand side the EnSite NavX™ visualization of the fractionation index. The same information is provided in the visualization on the right hand side by the visualization implementation of this work. There is a noticeable difference between both visualizations. The visualization method used in this work colors only small areas around measurement locations. All other locations where there is no information available will be displayed in grey. The EnSite NavX™ visualization instead has a large interpolation width so that the atria will be colored fully with only a few measurements.

Part III

Clinical Applications & Trials

11

Analysis of Coronary Sinus Signals

During nearly every electrophysiological examination a catheter is placed in the coronary sinus (CS). The catheter located in the CS can be placed stable over several hours. It is used to give information of the status of the atria during a catheter ablation. Thus, the signals recorded from this catheter can be used to analyze the organization during different atrial rhythms. Bipolar recordings were performed in the coronary sinus with a straight 8-pole catheter. The catheter is composed of 4 pairs of electrodes. The inter-electrode spacing of a pair is 2 mm and the spacing between pairs is 5 mm. The signals were sampled with 1 kHz and each signal has a length of 60 seconds. Only signals that were steady for the whole recording period have been taken into account. Recordings were performed during sinus rhythm, atrial flutter, and atrial fibrillation. In addition to the atrial signals the surface ECG has been recorded as reference. In this section a method is introduced that can analyze the regularity of signal patterns occurring during sinus rhythm, atrial flutter and atrial fibrillation. First, signal patterns for each rhythm are extracted. On these patterns a PCA is applied to cluster the patterns.

11.1 Segmenting & Clustering

All signals are recorded during EP studies and were preprocessed in the manner described in section 4.4. After removing high frequency noise and baseline wander, the atrial signals are divided into patterns reflecting atrial activity. Each lead of the CS catheter is processed on its own. To detect atrial activity, the absolute maximum amplitude is searched and the signal within 50 ms before and after the maximum is declared as a pattern. This region is marked as processed and the next absolute maximum is searched. The process stops if no further maxima are found or an amplitude threshold of 0.14 mV is reached. After that, all patterns are normalized and aligned to their maximum. With these patterns a data matrix $\mathbf{D}$ of size $N \times M$ is build, where N is the number of found patterns and M is the pattern length (here 100 ms).

$$\mathbf{D} = [\text{Pattern}_1, \ldots, \text{Pattern}_N]^T \tag{11.1}$$

On this data matrix a principle component analysis (PCA) is performed to reduce the number of patterns and to detect structure in the relation between the patterns. On basis of the first 5 principle components (PC) then a hierarchical clustering is performed. The first five eigenvalues in general contain more than 85% of the signals' variance, so it is suitable to use only the first five principle components for the clustering process. The purpose of clustering is to identify groups of data in the PCA space. Similar patterns will be transformed into the same regions in the PCA space. To find clusters, the city block distance d (11.2) for each pair of points (r,s) in the PCA space is calculated and a hierarchical cluster tree is build.

$$d_{rs} = \sum_{j=1}^{n} |x_{rj} - x_{sj}| \tag{11.2}$$

The cluster tree groups the data points according to their city block distance into clusters. All found clusters will be grouped successively into bigger clusters. To find the best cluster representation of the patterns, the cluster tree is cut manually such that the number of patterns is not exploding and the different patterns are separated into different clusters. Finally, the PC scores for each cluster are transformed back into the time domain.

11.2 Results of Coronary Sinus Analysis

To get an impression of the chaotic condition during atrial fibrillation, electrograms recorded in the coronary sinus are compared during sinus rhythm, atrial flutter, and atrial fibrillation. Active parts in the EGM are cut out, aligned to their maximum, and a PCA is performed. In the PCA space a clustering is performed afterwards. All signals have been preprocessed (sec. 4.4), but the ventricular far field has not been removed.

Figure 11.1 depicts the electrograms recorded during sinus rhythm. The atrial as well as the ventricular activity is clearly to be seen. When performing the clustering in the PCA space in each lead two clusters are found. One cluster corresponds

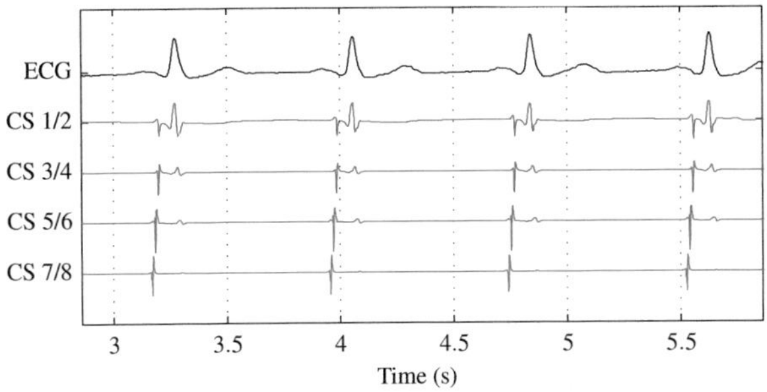

Fig. 11.1: Coronary sinus signals during sinus rhythm.

to the VFF and the other to atrial activity. The results of the clustering are depicted in figure 11.2. On the left hand side the results for lead CS 3/4 are shown and on the right hand side the results for lead CS 5/6. The upper line depicts the PCA space spanned by the first three principle components and the PCA representation of the patterns. The identified clusters are colored in cyan and red. The lower line shows the clustered patterns.

In case of sinus rhythm always two kind of clusters were found (fig. 11.2). Cluster 1 corresponds to the atrial signal and cluster 2, correlating to the QRS complex, represents the ventricular far field. Both signals are in regular rhythm corresponding to the heart rhythm measured on the surface. The number per interval of atrial signals and VFF corresponds to the calculated heart rate. From lead CS 1/2 over lead CS 3/4 and CS 5/6 to lead CS 7/8 the ventricular far field is getting smaller and is often not to be seen in lead CS 7/8 (fig. 11.1). The shape of patterns is very regular and there is no spread in shape.

Figure 11.3 depicts electrograms during atrial flutter. Compared to figure 11.1 it is obvious that the atrial frequency as well as the ventricular frequency is increased. The coronary sinus excitation is doubled compared to the ECG. This is called 2-1 transition, meaning that only each second atrial activation leads to a ventricular excitation. Also the VFF and each second atrial activity nearly coincide and can not be separated easily.

This is also reflected by the number of clusters observed. During atrial flutter there were mostly two kinds of signals. The first cluster of signals corresponds to the pure atrial excitation. The second cluster is a combination of atrial signals and VFF. After removing the ventricular far field from each pattern of the second clus-

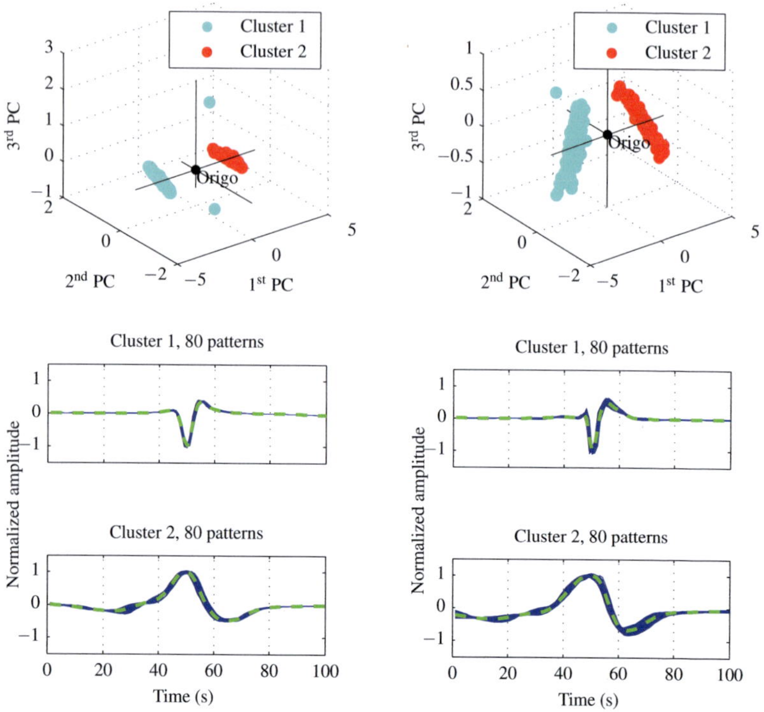

Fig. 11.2: Clustering results for the case of SR. Clustering was performed on leads CS 3/4 (left) and CS 5/6 (right). The green dashed line depicts the mean pattern of each cluster.

ter and performing another clustering, the first and second cluster are combined in the majority of cases. Compared with sinus rhythm the quantity of atrial patterns is more than doubled and there is a greater variation in shape. The patterns typically do not match as good as they do in sinus rhythm. So, aligning the patterns to the maximum peak sometimes fails and the misaligned patterns will produce outlier or will be found in a third cluster.

The electrograms for the case of atrial fibrillation are depicted in figure 11.5. It can be seen that it is not as easy to separate activity in the CS signals. Also the ventricular rhythm is irregular, which is evident from the ECG. During atrial fibrillation there is no such straight organization as found in the first two cases. The

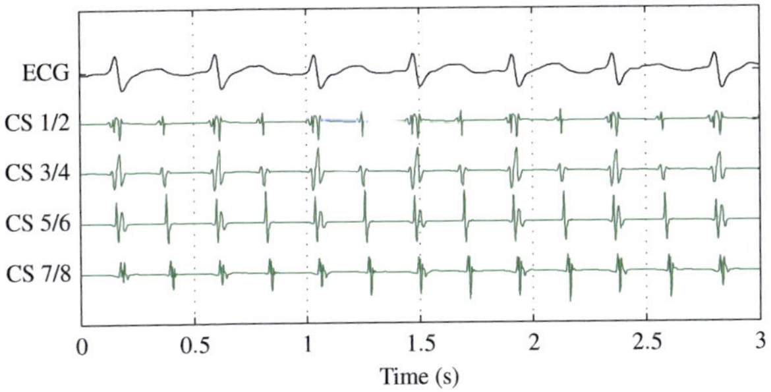

Fig. 11.3: Coronary sinus signals during atrial flutter.

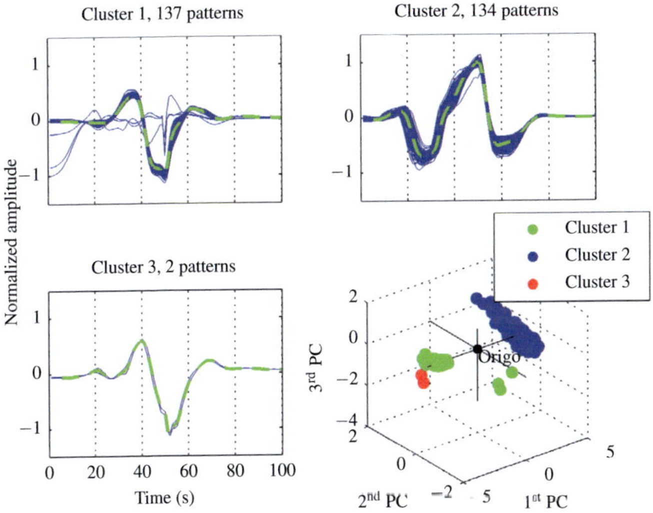

Fig. 11.4: Clustering results for the case of atrial flutter. Clustering was performed on lead CS 3/4. The green dashed line depicts the mean pattern of each cluster.

number of patterns and the number of clusters is increasing (fig. 11.6 and 11.7). Although some clusters look similar, there are noticeable differences in the shape of such signals (fig. 11.6). Also the spread of the shape for each cluster is increasing strongly. This is reflected in the PCA space, too. The data is scattered around the origin of ordinates and the distances between clusters is decreasing. This ex-

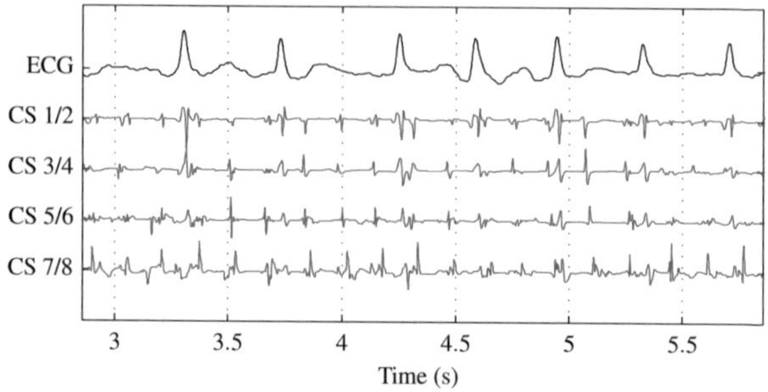

Fig. 11.5: Coronary sinus signals during atrial fibrillation.

amination was applied on data of different patients, that were sent to hospital for catheter ablation. Table 11.1 gives an overview of the found cluster for each patient and each atrial rhythm.

Table 11.1: Found number of clusters for each case. The cycle length is calculated from the number of patterns and the signal length.

Case No.	SR	AFlut	AF
1	2	2	15
2	2	2	14
3	2	2	20
4	2	2	12
5	2	2	22
$\overline{No_{Pattern}}$	80	268	450
$\overline{\text{cycle length}}$ (ms)	750	224	133

When heart rhythm evolves from sinus rhythm via atrial flutter to AF the number of clusters increases from 2 to approximately 17 for each lead, which means that the range of variation of patterns is getting larger. In addition, the organization of the signals is decreasing. In sinus rhythm atrial excitation is always followed by ventricular excitation. During atrial flutter not every atrial excitation will lead to a ventricular excitation. According to the atrial frequency only each second or third excitation will be trespassed to the ventricles. During AF theres is no correlation between atrial and ventricular activity. The ventricles act independent from the atria. This means that the VFF is decoupled from the atrial excitation. This is also

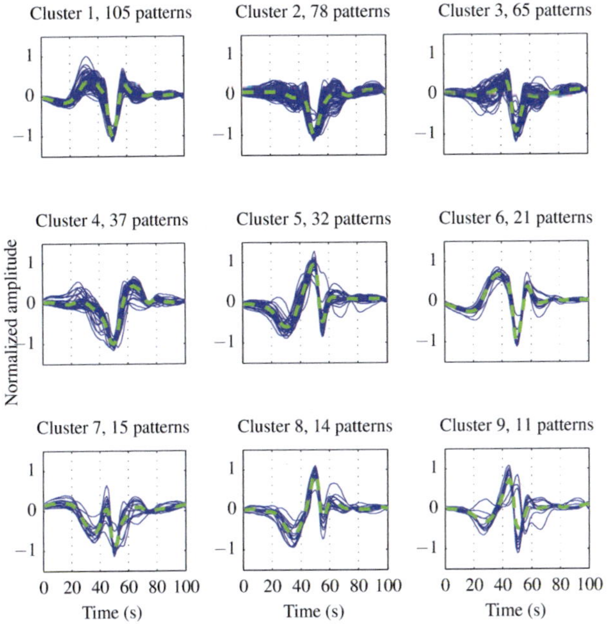

Fig. 11.6: Clustering results for the case of atrial fibrillation. Clustering was performed on lead CS 1/2. 14 cluster were found, but only the first 9 cluster are depicted. The green dashed line depicts the mean pattern of each cluster.

backed by the observation, that in case of AF, the observed patterns vary heavily in shape. This implies, that during AF there is no regularity in atrial activity. On the other hand, comparing the mean patterns, there is a recognizable similarity between some patterns. This implies, that AF is not that chaotic as assumed. The introduced method can be used to measure and display the increasing disarrangement of the excitation propagation from sinus rhythm to AF in an objective and quantitative way.

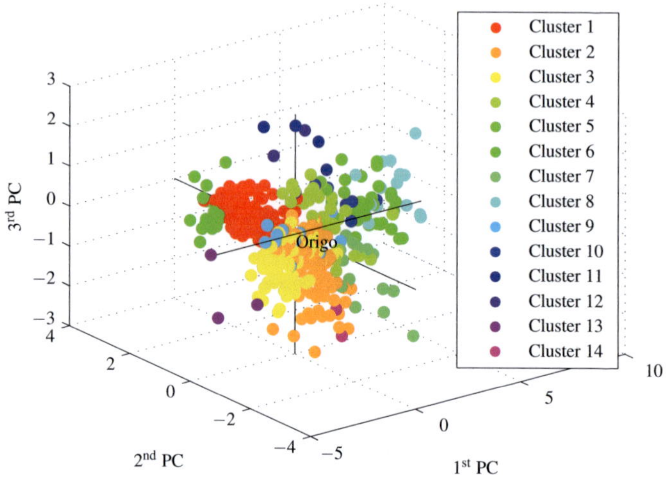

Fig. 11.7: PCA representation of the patterns during atrial fibrillation. PCA space spanned by the first three principle components.

12

Analyzing the Influence of Pulmonary Vein Isolation

12.1 Clinical Issue & Method

Catheter ablation of persistent atrial fibrillation is discussed controversially [46, 101]. The most promising strategy at the moment is the stepwise approach consisting of pulmonary vein isolation (PVI), ablation of complex fractionated electrograms (CFAE) and linear lesions [142]. Effects of the single steps are still unclear. To show the effect of PVI on the defractionation of the left atrium, CFAEmean maps were analyzed before and after PVI. Furthermore, maps that show the distribution of CFAE classes, NLEO energy, and activity ratio have been computed to confirm the outcome of commercial mapping systems.
Data was collected from 27 patients sent to hospital for catheter ablation suffering from AF. For each patient CFAEmean maps of the left atrium were performed before and after PVI using the EnSite NavX™ system. Both maps were recorded during atrial fibrillation. Data was transferred and reconstructed by the methods presented in this work. To point not only the outcome of one descriptor, three more descriptors have been chosen to analyze the effect of PVI. Besides the mean fractionation of an electrogram (CFAEmean), CFAE classification derived from the fuzzy decision tree, the energy calculated with the non-linear energy operator, and the activity ratio gained from segmenting EGMs have been analyzed.

12.2 Results of the Influence of PVI

The main problem while analyzing descriptor maps recorded at different times, is that the measurements positions are commonly not the same and also the number of measurements vary heavily. Furthermore, all data was recorded during daily practice in the EP lab, what makes accurate recordings difficult. Thus, interpreting mean, median or other measures of distributions might be ambiguous as some regions might be over- and other regions underrepresented. Hence, a single number will not give a good conclusion. The generated maps were evaluated by physicians retrospectively. The following results and discussions hold true for all recorded data, but only one case is depicted exemplarily in figures 12.1 and 12.2. White

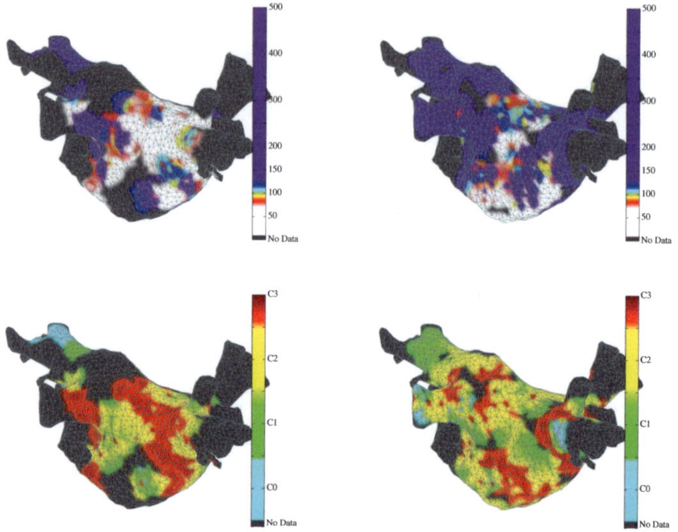

Fig. 12.1: Maps recorded before (left) and after (right) PVI. Shown are the distributions for the CFAEmean (upper) and the extracted CFAE classes (lower).

areas in the CFAEmean map reflect high fractionation, whereas purple areas are considered to represent healthy tissue (fig. 12.1). Comparing the CFAEmean map before and after PVI, one can state, that size and number of high fractionated (white) areas are decreasing. Coinciding, the size and number of not fractionated (purple) areas increase. That implies, that after PVI less fractionation is visible and, therefore, less CFAEs can be detected. PVI isolates the triggers originating within the pulmonary veins. Preventing the excitation originating from these triggers to reach the atrium, leads to a undistorted view on the atrial substrate and the fibrillating tissue within the atrium. The PVI has also an effect on the distribution of CFAE classes. There are more areas assigned to CFAE class C3 (continuous activity) before than after PVI. After PVI there are lot of more areas assigned to CFAE class C1 and C2. These classes represent more regular activity. Comparing the distribution of CFAE classes with the CFAEmean, mostly high fractionation areas correspond with CFAE class C3. In some casses continuous activity will also be found in not fractionated areas (chap. 13). The energy calculated with a non-linear energy operator shows lower energy values for the map after PVI (fig. 12.2). This might correspond with the decreasing number of high fractionated electrograms. At the moment, there is no plain relation between ischemia and energy, respectively the amplitude, of an EGM as it is defined in the ventricles. Thus, interpreting a signal's energy has to be done carefully. Nevertheless, higher energy values correspond with higher fractionation. Finally, the effect of PVI can be shown with activity ratio, too. The activity ratio is a measure for continuous activity. Continuous activity is always high fractionated activity, but high fractionation does not imply continuous activity. Before PVI there is more continuous activity to be seen (activity ratio tends to be 1) as after PVI.

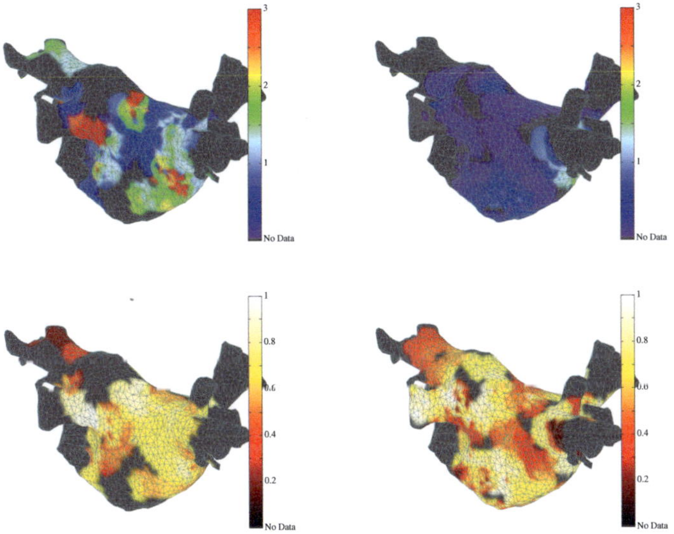

Fig. 12.2: Maps recorded before (left) and after (right) PVI. Shown are the distributions for the NLEO-based energy (upper) and the activity ratio (lower).

So, the effect of isolating the pulmonary veins and preventing pulmonary activity from reaching the atrium could be shown with different independent descriptors. Even in patients with persistent AF the isolation of the pulmonary veins can reduce the substrate for atrial fibrillation. Therefore, PVI should be the first step in a stepwise approach.
Pulmonary vein isolation alone does affect the mean fractionation, CFAE class distribution, signals' energy, and activity ratio in the left atrium in patients with persistent atrial fibrillation. This has implications for ablation strategies for persistent atrial fibrillation.

13

Continuous Activity with High Fractionation during AF

13.1 Clinical Issue & Method

Despite the knowledge received from clinical studies and trials, the exact mechanism of AF is still unknown. Especially, the importance of ablating complex fractionated atrial electrograms (CFAEs) is discussed [143–145]. Continuous activity has been reported to be a promising target for terminating AF. However, there is at the moment no supporting commercial algorithm to detect continuous activity. Thus, the physicians are preselecting interesting areas in the atria by the automated fractionation index algorithm. In areas of high fractionation then electrograms with continuous activity are searched.

It is common practice to use 3D maps of the fractionation of signals while ablating persistent AF [65,136]. The EnSite NavX™ algorithm can localize areas with high fractionation (CFAEs), but high fractionation areas not necessarily overlap with continuous activity signals. Therefore, selective ablation of continuous activity remains operator dependent. Based on the information gained from the 3D maps and the analysis of the measured EGMs physicians plan the ablation strategy. The setup of the commonly used CFAEmean index (sec. 7.5.1) is very dependent on the fashion of each physician. Commonly, the CFAEmean map is divided into three regions. High fractionated EGMs are supposed to have a mean cycle length smaller than 120 ms (R1). Regular activity is supposed to have a cycle length of larger than 200 ms (R3). The region in between (R2) is a border zone with CFAEs more or less important to the ablation process.

The CFEAmean conveys the impression, that the fractionation in region R1 and R3 are homogenous. As CFAEmean does not necessarily reflect the occurrence of continuous activity, this homogeneity might be not that uniform. Together with physicians from Städtisches Klinikum Karlsruhe the divergence in these different

regions with independent descriptors was analyzed. Additional descriptors may provide new information in understanding the AF substrate.
In the prospect of this study 7800 EGMs from 27 patients suffering from AF were retrospectively analyzed. CFAEmean maps were recorded during electrophysiolocical examinations by use of the EnSite NavX™ software (St. Jude Medical, St. Paul, Mn, USA). Stable rhythms at different regions of the left atrium are recorded with conventional catheters using the EnGuide-System. The automated algorithm of the EnSite NavX™ system is used to identify fractionated electrograms. A list of settings for the EnSite NavX™ algorithm are made as usual by the physicians (P-P sensitivity = 0.04 mV, electrogram detection: –dV/dt, refractory = 40 ms, segment length = 5 s, etc.). For each recorded region the automated algorithm delivers a fractionation index (CFAEmean) based on the cycle length of distinguishable local activities in one electrogram and the (x,y,z)-coordinates of the electrode location.
For each recorded electrogram the NLEO-based energy (NLEOenergy), activity ratio (AR), mean length of active segments (MLAS), and the number of active segments (NoAS) are computed. The definition for all descriptors can be found in chapter 7. The distribution for each descriptor in the specified regions is computed on the patient data (fig. 13.1). The results are visualized by use of boxplot representation and the probability density function is shown, to give a more accurate view on the maximum dispersion of the distribution. The PDF is estimated with a kernel density function (gaussian normal). Additionally, the distribution for each descriptor on the patient specific atrium can be visualized (fig. 13.2).

13.2 Results of Characterizing Continuous Activity

The maximum value of NLEOenergy is decreasing from region R1 to region R2 and R3. The median values are significantly different on a 5% niveau. Also the distribution is shifted to smaller values, which can be seen by the estimated PDF. The distributions of region R2 and R3 are nearly equal (fig. 13.1).
The evaluation of the activity ratio (AR) showed a slight change in the PDF. Region R1 and R2 are not significantly different, but region R3 has a significantly larger median, whereas the maxima and minima are not changing. The mean length of active segments (MLAS) is increasing from region R1 to region R3. This is reflected by the increasing maximum value as well as the increasing median. The PDF is changing from a bulgy to a more long-drawn-out dispersion. Finally, com-

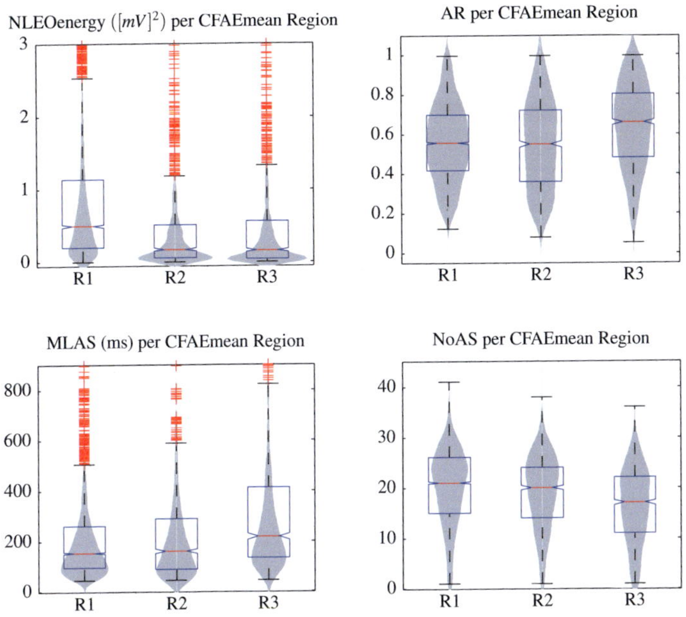

Fig. 13.1: Descriptor distributions for the specified CFAEmean regions. It can be seen, that the CFAEmean regions are not homogenous, when taking a different look at them. R1: 0 – 120 ms, R2: 120 – 200 ms, R3: >200 ms.

pared to the MLAS, the number of active segments (NoAS) behaves the other way around. Maximum values and medians are decreasing from region R1 to region R3. Here, also the boxes, representing the first and third quartile, are moving towards smaller values.

While ablating AF the physician is searching for high fractionated and continuous activity. Commonly he/she is supported by commercial software like EnSite NavX™. A CFAEmean map will separate high fractionated from less fractionated EGMs. A mean cycle length with values smaller than 120 ms is considered as high fractionated and a mean cycle length larger than 200 ms as regular. But, high fractionation areas cover not necessarily continuous active signals.

Comparing the new introduced descriptors for the specified regions, one can state, that the regions are not as homogenous as expected, when only taking the CFAE-

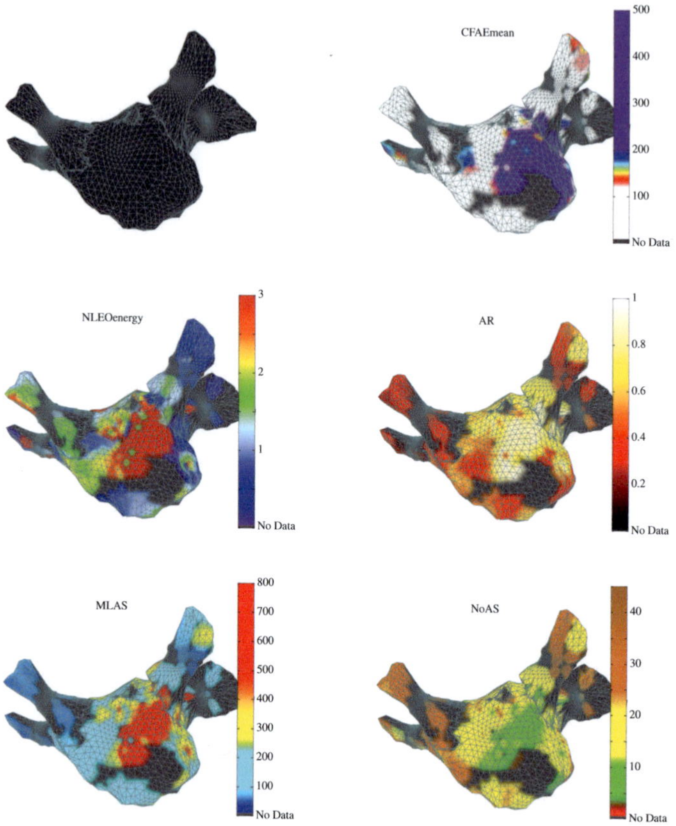

Fig. 13.2: Visualization of the presented descriptors on a patient specific map of the left atrium during atrial fibrillation. Areas where no EGMs have been measured are colored in dark grey. The upper left picture depicts the patient specific atrial geometry recorded during an electrophysiological study. Region R1 corresponds to the white areas in the CFEAmean map (upper right), region R3 to the purple area and region R2 to the remaining colors.

mean into account. Region R1 is assumed to be the most fractionated region, but activity ratio is not changing significantly from region R1 to region R2. Similar findings result from NoAS and MLAS. Only the NLEOenergy gives a significant difference between region R1 and R2. Fig. 13.2 depicts the descriptor distribution of a single case. It can be seen, that additional information can improve the findings from the CFAEmean map and can give a more detailed view on CFAEs. Taking a closer look at CFAEs and using more than one information gained from these signals is advisable. The presentation of new and additional information gained from the CFAEs can improve the knowledge about atrial fibrillation substrate and therefore, lead to improved ablation success.

14

Conclusion

The scope of this project was to investigate atrial electrograms during atrial fibrillation to improve the understanding and knowledge of these signals. The main interest here was the investigation of complex fractionated atrial electrograms (CFAEs). First, the ventricular far field has been analyzed and removed from atrial signals. This was achieved with a principle component based algorithm. It could be shown, that the presence of ventricular far fields will lead to ambiguous investigations of the atrial activity. The applied method removes not only the superimposed ventricular activity, but also recovers the atrial activity. Thus, this method is a basic step for further analysis of atrial signals without superimposition. Next, a segmentation into active and inactive parts was done by a non-linear energy operator with adaptive thresholding. The frequency as well as the amplitude are taken into account to detect active parts. The detected active segments represent the interesting parts of atrial activity during atrial fibrillation. This segmentation reflects the physician's view on signals and is a basis of finding attributes for these signals. To get a deeper understanding of fractionated signals during atrial fibrillation, different descriptors have been introduced, that characterize and measure attributes. That way new signal representations were found for time domain, frequency domain, and phase space. Additional characteristics were encountered by wavelet-based, NLEO-based, and statistics-based methods. All introduced descriptors reflected the influence of diverging atrial rhythms on the electrogram. Also different types of fractionated electrograms lead to different representation by the descriptors.

At the moment one main strategy to find the arrhythmogenic atrial substrate is the analysis of the mean fractionation of an electrogram. Nevertheless, this covers only one part of the definition of CFAEs. Continuous activity is reported a successful ablation target, but will not be detected. Additional descriptors like CFAE classes, activity ratio, or the energy of an electrogram will detect continuous activity and provide, therefore, valuable information. The presence of different types of fractionated electrograms during atrial fibrillation is accepted in the medical community, but they are disputed and their definition is ambiguous. Nevertheless, they have been reported to play an important role during catheter ablation. A fuzzy decision tree has been implemented that can distinguish between different kinds of reported CFAEs. This classifier is a combination of a classical decision tree with fuzzy-logic. In addition to a classification result a certainty for this result is given. Thus, the reliability of the given result can be estimated. In the scope of this work, the fuzzy decision tree can give objective decisions, that can be a guidance for physicians or can help to find a more universal definition of CFAEs. A second classifier was presented to detect signals that have been measured with insufficient catheter contact to the endocardium. Catheter contact is important to measure reliable signals as well as to set transmural lesions while ablation. The decision tree shown in this work, implements the physicians' observation of the changing morphology of an electrogram when loosing catheter contact. Furthermore, a computer simulation of a catheter and an atrial tissue patch was realized to generate electrograms with different catheter orientations to the endocardium. This way the physicians' observations could be proven and extended. The new gained information is visualized on patient specific 3D models of the atria. Thus, the information is presented in a way physicians are used to. This lowers the doubts about unknown methods and provides a quick evaluation of new descriptors and comparison to regularly used descriptors. The interpolation width in commercially used mapping systems is adjustable. Commonly, the interpolation width is set to high values, to get a colored map with only a few measurements. This leads hardly to reliable representation of the arrhythmia. Against this, the 3D maps introduced in the scope of this work, have a very small interpolation and reflect rather the real state of knowledge of the arrhythmia.

Finally, clinical applications of the presented methods were realized. In a first investigation the regularity of atrial activity recorded in the coronary sinus was examined. Signals recorded from the coronary sinus catheter are used as reference for the state of the atrium. Signal patterns were extracted for sinus rhythm, atrial flutter, and atrial fibrillation. It could be shown that the regularity is decreasing when the heart rhythm evolves from sinus rhythm to atrial fibrillation, but the pattern distribution is not as chaotic as expected. The variance of the amplitudes' morphology is increasing, however, there is recognizable similarity between some mean patterns. This approach can be used, to measure and display increasing disarrangement of atrial patterns in an objective and quantitative way. The proceeding during ablation of persistent atrial fibrillation is still discussed. With the introduced methods applied on data of 27 patients, it could be shown that pulmonary vein isolation influences the representation of the atrial substrate. 3D maps that display the mean fractionation have been compared to energy maps, activity ratio maps, and maps that display the distribution of recognized CFAE classes. Maps have been recorded before and after pulmonary vein isolation. All map representations showed, that pulmonary vein isolation decreases the complexity and divergence of the single descriptors and, thus, pulmonary vein isolation alone does affect and can reduce the substrate for atrial fibrillation. Continuous activity has been reported to be a promising target for terminating atrial fibrillation. However, there is at the moment no way to detect electrograms with continuous activity automatically. The distribution for several descriptors in regularly used CFAEmean regions were computed. It could be shown, that CFAEmean index does not reflect the occurrence of continuous activity. So, taking a closer look at CFAEs and using more than one information gained from these signals is advisable and could lead to promising ablation outcomes.

All developed methods could be used for online analysis of the electrograms recorded in the EP lab. Implementing these methods into electro-anatomical mapping systems, will give a fast analysis and provide new information of high diagnostic value.

Catheter ablation is a lead and on-top technology in the cure of atrial arrhythmias. Nevertheless, mechanisms of the underlying disorder and the origin of complex fractionated atrial electrograms are discussed controversially and take part in clinical investigations. The developed methods can be a step forward in understanding atrial fibrillation and CFAEs.

In summary, it was shown that additional representation of complex fractionated atrial electrograms leads to more information of the underlying arrhythmia. Investigating not only the fractionation of an electrogram by evaluating the cycle length, but also interpreting information obtained from several new descriptors could improve the ablation outcome. Providing the physician with additional valuable information about fractionated electrograms will, hopefully, shorten ablation time, improve the success rate of the procedure and will decrease the number of recurrence. Thus, the general treatment costs could be reduced and the patients' burden will be lowered.

A follow-up project of this work is granted by the *German Research Foundation* with the title "Merkmalsextraktion und Klassifizierung komplex fraktionierter atrialer Elektrogramme (CFAEs)" ("Feature Extraction and Classification of Complex Fractionated Atrial Electrograms (CFAEs)"). This project will be a joint research project of Städtisches Klinikum Karlsruhe and the Institute of Biomedical Engineering. Aim of this new project is to carry on the fundamental investigations presented in this thesis and to start clinical studies.

Part IV

Appendix

A

Boxplots of all Introduced Descriptors

A.1 CFAE Class Descriptors

In the following all boxplots of the descriptors computed on the database introduced in section 4.3.1 are displayed. The descriptors are used to distinguish between different CFAE classes. All together 429 EGMs have been classified. They are split into 144 EGMs in CFAE class C0, 84 in CFAE class C1, 148 in CFAE class C2, and 53 in CFAE class C3. In addition to each boxplot, the probability density function for each distribution (PDF) is depicted, to give a more accurate view on the maximum dispersion of the distribution. The PDF is estimated based on a Gaussian kernel function. The full naming for the descriptors can be seen in table 8.3.

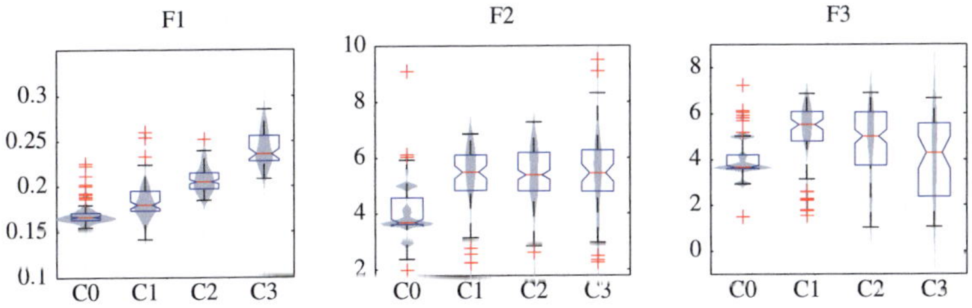

Fig. A.1: Boxplot visualization and PDF for the different descriptors computed on the CFAE classes database.

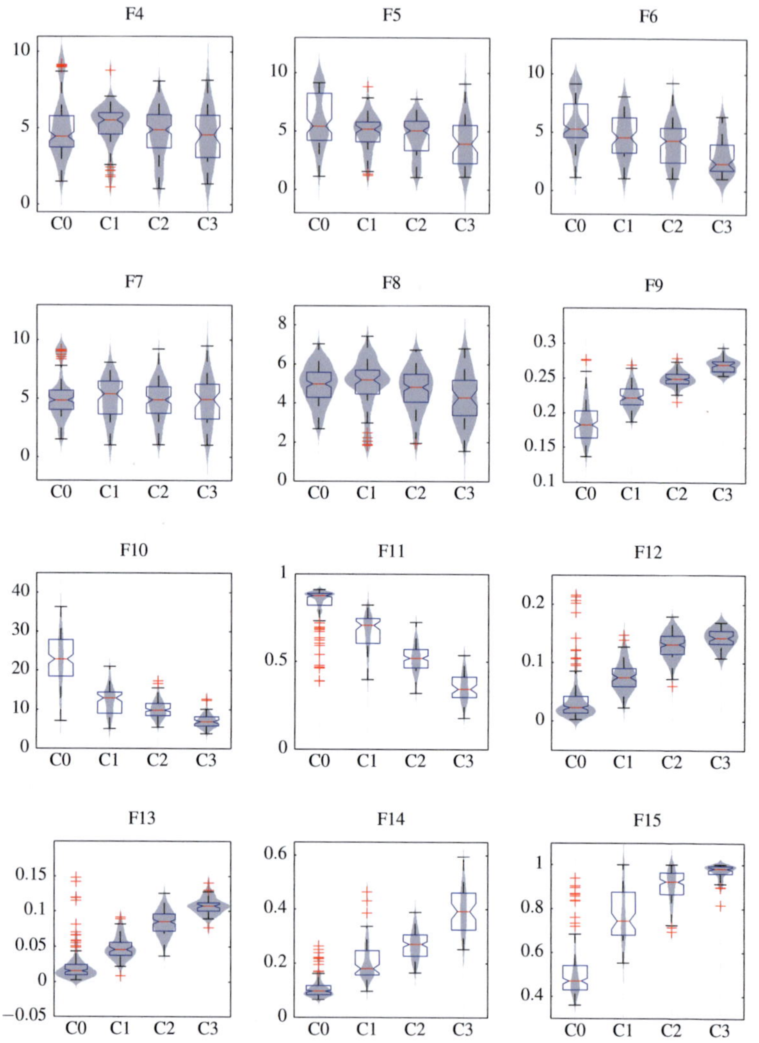

Fig. A.2: Boxplot visualization and PDF for the different descriptors computed on the CFAE classes database.

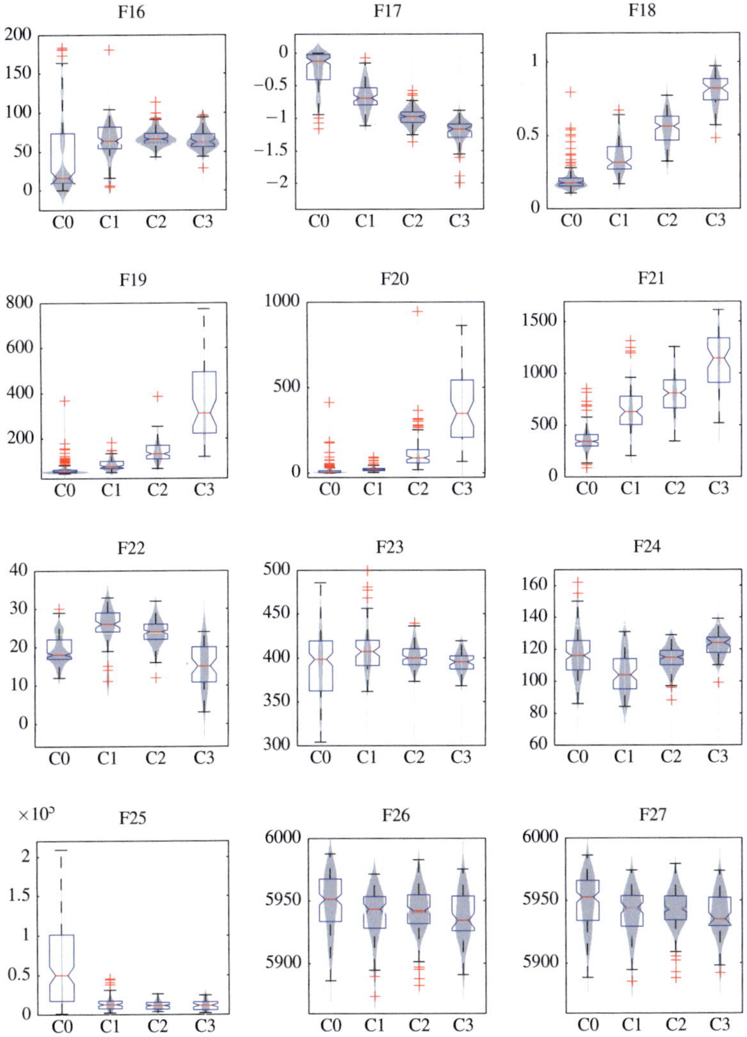

Fig. A.3: Boxplot visualization and PDF for the different descriptors computed on the CFAE classes database.

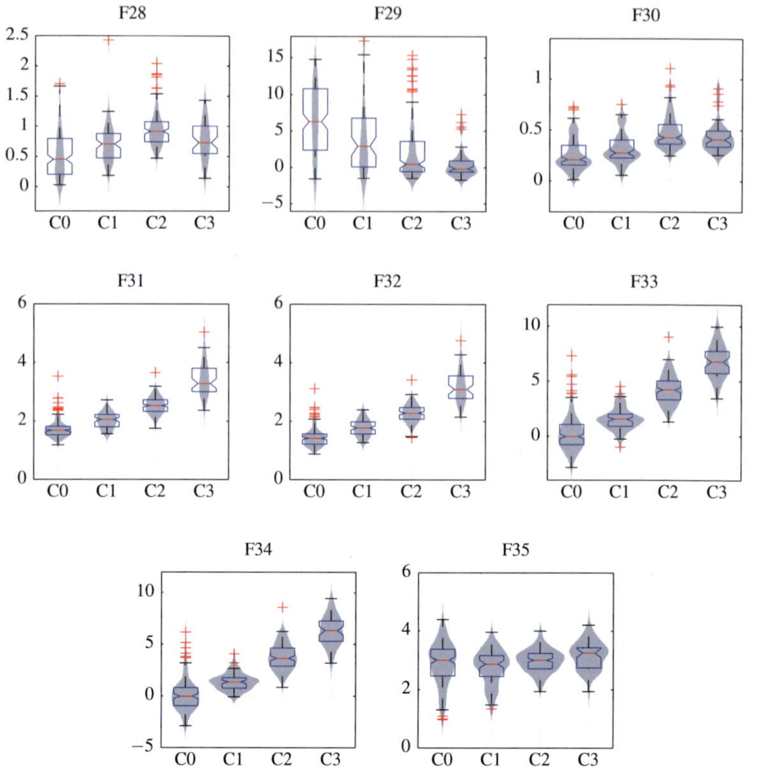

Fig. A.4: Boxplot visualization and PDF for the different descriptors computed on the CFAE classes database.

A.2 Contact vs. Non-contact Descriptors

In the following all boxplots of the descriptors computed on the database introduced in section 4.3.3 are displayed. The descriptors are used to distinguish between contact and non-contact electrograms. 149 contact EGMs and 107 non-contact EGMs are evaluated. In addition to each boxplot, the probability density function for each distribution (PDF) is depicted, to give a more accurate view on the maximum dispersion of the distribution. The PDF is estimated based on a Gaussian kernel function. The full naming for the descriptors can be seen in table 9.2.

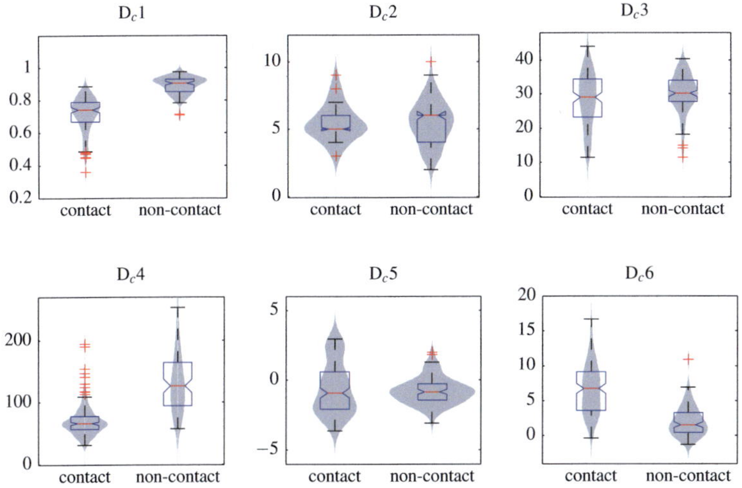

Fig. A.5: Boxplot visualization and PDF for the different descriptors computed on the contact/non-contact database.

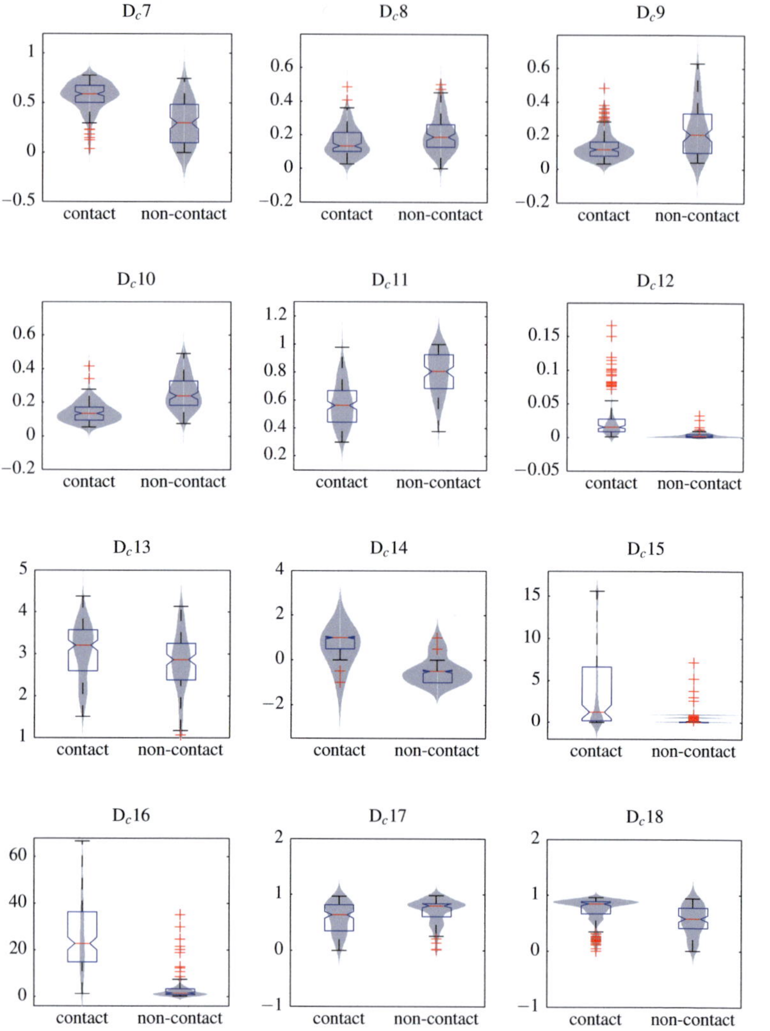

Fig. A.6: Boxplot visualization and PDF for the different descriptors computed on the contact/non-contact database.

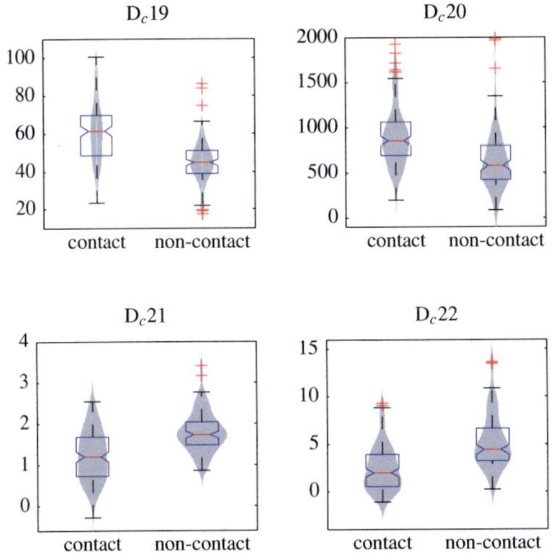

Fig. A.7: Boxplot visualization and PDF for the different descriptors computed on the contact/non-contact database.

B

Simulated Electrograms

In the following all signals resulting from the simulation introduced in chapter 9 are displayed. First, the results gained from the simulations with a point-electrode are depicted. Distances between the catheter and the endocardium of 0 mm, 0.1 mm, 1 mm, and 2 mm are realized. Because of the limited size of the simulation environment, a distance of 2 mm for catheter position 5 could not be realized.

Next, the simulation results from a modeled catheter are shown. Distances between the catheter and the endocardium of 0 mm, 0.1 mm, 0.5 mm, 1 mm, and 2 mm are realized. Because of the limited size of the simulation environment, a distance of 2 mm for catheter position 5 could not be realized.

B.1 Point-electrode Catheter

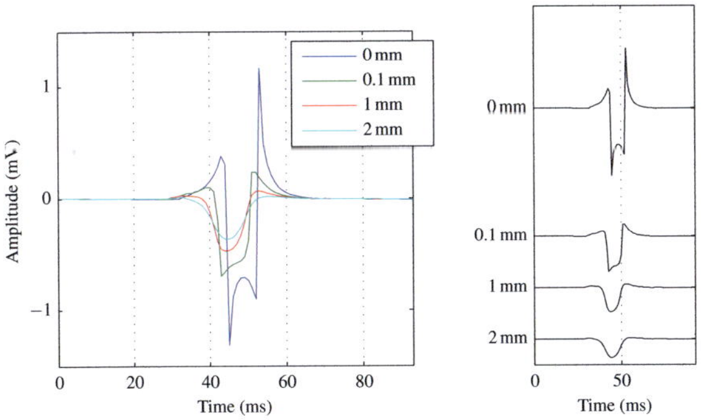

Fig. B.1: Simulated EGMs received from a point-electrode catheter in position 1 (tab. 9.1).

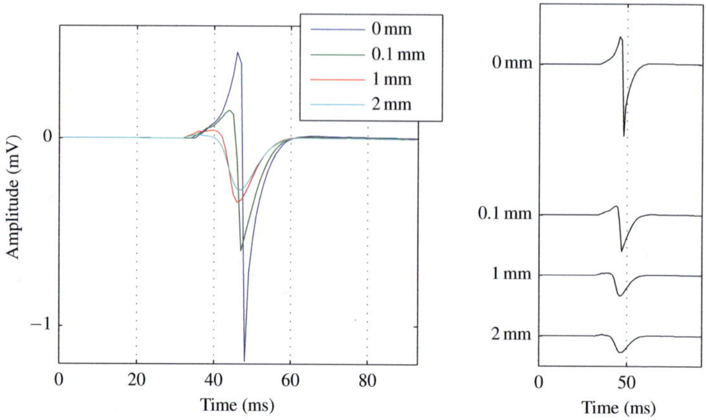

Fig. B.2: Simulated EGMs received from a point-electrode catheter in position 2 (tab. 9.1).

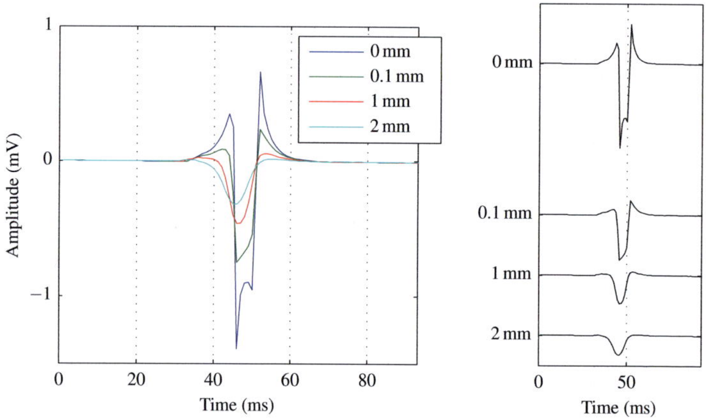

Fig. B.3: Simulated EGMs received from a point-electrode catheter in position 3 (tab. 9.1).

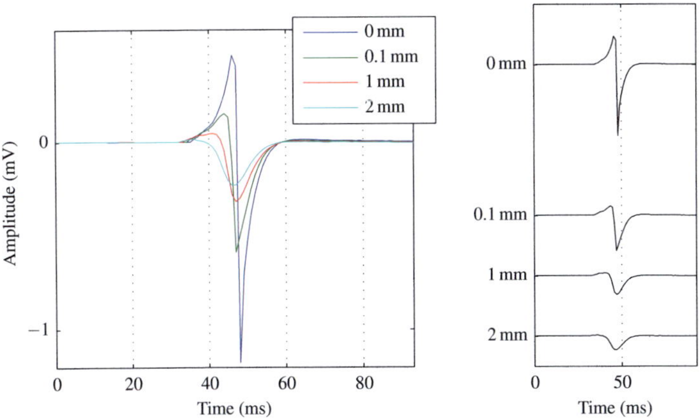

Fig. B.4: Simulated EGMs received from a point-electrode catheter in position 4 (tab. 9.1).

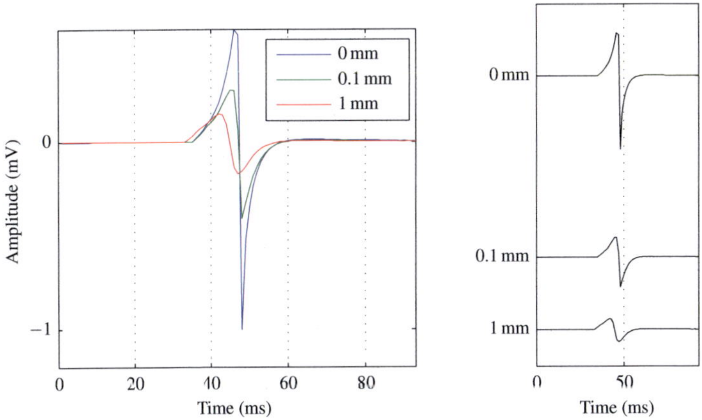

Fig. B.5: Simulated EGMs received from a point-electrode catheter in position 5 (tab. 9.1).

B.2 Modeled Catheter

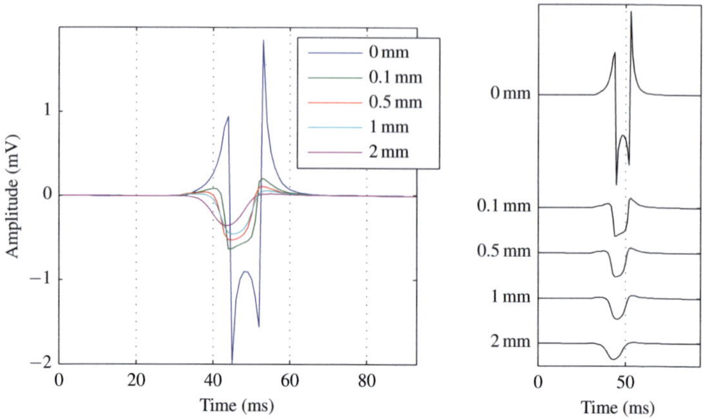

Fig. B.6: Simulated EGMs received from a modeled catheter in position 1 (tab. 9.1).

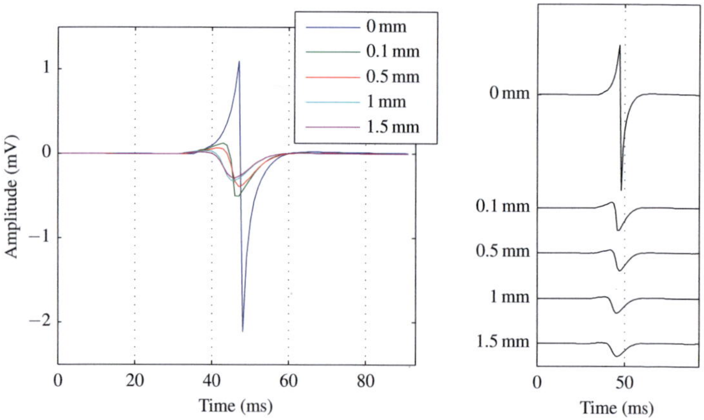

Fig. B.7: Simulated EGMs received from a modeled catheter in position 2 (tab. 9.1).

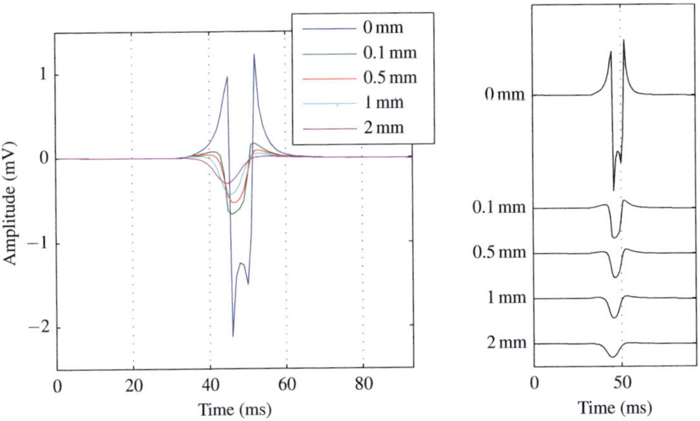

Fig. B.8: Simulated EGMs received from a modeled catheter in position 3 (tab. 9.1).

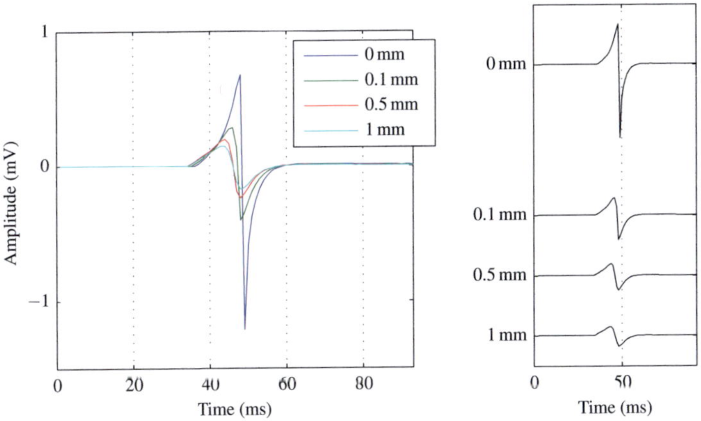

Fig. B.9: Simulated EGMs received from a modeled catheter in position 5 (tab. 9.1).

References

1. V. Fuster, L. E. Rydén, D. S. Cannom, H. J. Crijns, A. B. Curtis, K. A. Ellenbogen, J. L. Halperin, G. N. Kay, J.-Y. Le Huezey, J. E. Lowe, S. B. Olsson, E. N. Prystowsky, J. L. Tamargo, L. S. Wann, S. C. Smith, Jr, S. G. Priori, N. A. M. Estes, 3rd, M. D. Ezekowitz, W. M. Jackman, C. T. January, J. E. Lowe, R. L. Page, D. J. Slotwiner, W. G. Stevenson, C. M. Tracy, A. K. Jacobs, J. L. Anderson, N. Albert, C. E. Buller, M. A. Creager, S. M. Ettinger, R. A. Guyton, J. L. Halperin, J. S. Hochman, F. G. Kushner, E. M. Ohman, W. G. Stevenson, L. G. Tarkington, C. W. Yancy, and American College of Cardiology Foundation/American Heart Association Task Force, "2011 ACCF/AHA/HRS focused updates incorporated into the ACC/AHA/ESC 2006 guidelines for the management of patients with atrial fibrillation: A report of the American College of Cardiology Foundation/American Heart Association Task Force on practice guidelines," *Circulation*, vol. 123, pp. e269–367, Mar 2011.
2. Statistisches Bundesamt, *Diagnosedaten der Patienten und Patientinnen in Krankenhäusern (einschl. Sterbe- und Stundenfälle) 2010.* Statistisches Bundesamt, 2011.
3. R. F. Schmidt, G. Thews, and F. Lang, *Physiologie des Menschen.* Berlin; Heidelberg; New York: Springer, 2000.
4. S. Silbernagl and A. Despopoulos, *Taschenatlas Physiologie.* Thieme, 2007.
5. S. N. Oesterle, N. Reifart, E. Hauptmann, M. Hayase, and A. C. Yeung, "Percutaneous in situ coronary venous arterialization: Report of the first human catheter-based coronary artery bypass," *Circulation*, vol. 103, pp. 2539–43, May 2001.
6. J. Malmivuo and R. Plonsey, *Bioelectromagnetism. Principles and applications of bioelectric and biomagnetic fields.* New York Oxford: Oxford University Press, 1995.
7. A. Bolz and W. Urbaszek, *Technik in der Kardiologie: Eine interdisziplinäre Darstellung.* Berlin, Heidelberg: Springer, 2002.
8. E. Patterson and B. J. Scherlag, "Decremental Conduction in the Posterior and Anterior AV Nodal Inputs," *Journal of Interventional Cardiac Electrophysiology*, vol. 7, pp. 137–148, 2002.
9. F. Lang and P. Lang, *Basiswissen Physiologie.* Springer-Lehrbuch, Berlin, Heidelberg: Springer Medizin Verlag Heidelberg, 2007.
10. W. Einthoven, "Weiteres über das Elektrokardiogramm," *Pflügers Archiv*, vol. 122, pp. 517–584, 1908.
11. E. Goldberger, "A simple, indifferent, electrocardiographic electrode of zero potential and a technique of obtaining augmented, unipolar, extremity leads," *American Heart Journal*, vol. 23, pp. 483–492, 1942.

12. E. Goldberger, "The aVL, aVR, and aVF leads: A simplification of standard lead electrocardiography," *American Heart Journal*, vol. 24, pp. 378–396, 1942.
13. F. N. Wilson, A. G. Macleod, and P. S. Barker, "The potential variations produced by the heart beat at the apices of Einthoven," *American Heart Journal*, vol. 7, pp. 207–211, 1931.
14. F. N. Wilson, F. D. Johnston, A. G. Macleod, and P. S. Barker, "Electrocardiograms that represent the potential variations of a single electrode," *American Heart Journal*, vol. 9, pp. 447–458, 1934.
15. S. Ho and D. Sánchez-Quintana, "The importance of atrial structure and fibers," *Clinical Anatomy*, vol. 22, no. 1, pp. 52–63, 2009.
16. J. Neuzner and H. F. Pitschner, *Vorhofflimmern, Vorhofflattern: Aktuelle Diagnostik und Therapie*. Steinkopff, 2006.
17. H. Calkins, J. Brugada, D. Packer, R. Cappato, S. Chen, H. Crijns, R. Damiano, D. Davies, D. Haines, M. Haissaguerre, *et al.*, "HRS/EHRA/ECAS expert consensus statement on catheter and surgical ablation of atrial fibrillation: recommendations for personnel, policy, procedures and follow-up a report of the Heart Rhythm Society (HRS) task force on catheter and surgical ablation of atrial fibrillation. Developed in partnership with the European Heart Rhythm Association (EHRA) and the European Cardiac Arrhythmia Society (ECAS); in collaboration with the American College of Cardiology (ACC), American Heart Association (AHA), and the Society of Thoracic Surgeons (STS). Endorsed and approved by the governing bodies of the American College of Cardiology, the American Heart Association, the European Cardiac Arrhythmia Society, the European Heart Rhythm Association, the Society of Thoracic Surgeons, and the Heart Rhythm Society," *Heart Rhythm*, vol. 4, no. 6, pp. 816–861, 2007.
18. S. Levy, A. Camm, S. Saksena, E. Aliot, G. Breithardt, H. Crijns, W. Davies, N. Kay, E. Prystowsky, R. Sutton, *et al.*, "International consensus on nomenclature and classification of atrial fibrillation: A collaborative project of the Working Group on Arrhythmias and the Working Group on Cardiac Pacing of the European Society of Cardiology and the North American Society of Pacing and Electrophysiology," *Europace*, vol. 5, no. 2, p. 119, 2003.
19. D. G. Wyse and B. J. Gersh, "Atrial fibrillation: A perspective - Thinking inside and outside the box," *Circulation*, vol. 109, pp. 3089–95, Jun 2004.
20. A. J. Shah, X. Liu, A. S. Jadidi, and M. Haïssaguerre, "Early management of atrial fibrillation: from imaging to drugs to ablation," *Nat Rev Cardiol*, vol. 7, pp. 345–54, Jun 2010.
21. S. Stewart, C. Hart, D. Hole, and J. McMurray, "Population prevalence, incidence, and predictors of atrial fibrillation in the Renfrew/Paisley study," *British Medical Journal*, vol. 86, no. 5, p. 516, 2001.
22. S. Stewart, C. Hart, D. Hole, and J. McMurray, "A population-based study of the long-term risks associated with atrial fibrillation: 20-year follow-up of the Renfrew/Paisley study," *The American journal of medicine*, vol. 113, no. 5, pp. 359–364, 2002.
23. D. Lloyd-Jones, T. Wang, E. Leip, M. Larson, D. Levy, R. Vasan, R. D'Agostino, J. Massaro, A. Beiser, P. Wolf, *et al.*, "Lifetime risk for development of atrial fibrillation: The Framingham Heart Study," *Circulation*, vol. 110, no. 9, p. 1042, 2004.
24. J. Heeringa, D. van der Kuip, A. Hofman, J. Kors, G. van Herpen, B. Stricker, T. Stijnen, G. Lip, and J. Witteman, "Prevalence, incidence and lifetime risk of atrial fibrillation: the Rotterdam study," *European Heart Journal*, vol. 27, no. 8, p. 949, 2006.
25. P. Kirchhof, A. Auricchio, J. Bax, H. Crijns, J. Camm, H. Diener, A. Goette, G. Hindricks, S. Hohnloser, L. Kappenberger, *et al.*, "Outcome parameters for trials in atrial fibrillation: Executive sum-

mary," *European heart journal*, vol. 28, no. 22, p. 2803, 2007.

26. W. Kannel, R. Abbott, D. Savage, and P. McNamara, "Epidemiologic features of chronic atrial fibrillation: The Framingham study," *New England Journal of Medicine*, vol. 306, no. 17, p. 1018, 1982.
27. E. Benjamin, P. Wolf, R. D'Agostino, H. Silbershatz, W. Kannel, and D. Levy, "Impact of atrial fibrillation on the risk of death: The Framingham Heart Study," *Circulation*, vol. 98, no. 10, p. 946, 1998.
28. T. Wang, M. Larson, D. Levy, R. Vasan, E. Leip, P. Wolf, R. D'Agostino, J. Murabito, W. Kannel, and E. Benjamin, "Temporal relations of atrial fibrillation and congestive heart failure and their joint influence on mortality: The Framingham Heart Study," *Circulation*, vol. 107, no. 23, p. 2920, 2003.
29. W. Kannel, P. Wolf, E. Benjamin, and D. Levy, "Prevalence, incidence, prognosis, and predisposing conditions for atrial fibrillation: Population-based estimates.," *The American journal of cardiology*, vol. 82, no. 8A, p. 2N, 1998.
30. F. Khairallah, R. Ezzedine, L. Ganz, B. London, and S. Saba, "Epidemiology and determinants of outcome of admissions for atrial fibrillation in the United States from 1996 to 2001," *The American journal of cardiology*, vol. 94, no. 4, pp. 500–504, 2004.
31. J. Friberg, P. Buch, H. Scharling, N. Gadsbøll, and G. Jensen, "Rising rates of hospital admissions for atrial fibrillation," *Epidemiology*, pp. 666–672, 2003.
32. W. Wattigney, G. Mensah, and J. Croft, "Increasing trends in hospitalization for atrial fibrillation in the United States, 1985 through 1999: Implications for primary prevention," *circulation*, vol. 108, no. 6, p. 711, 2003.
33. S. Stewart, K. MacIntyre, M. MacLeod, A. Bailey, S. Capewell, and J. McMurray, "Trends in hospital activity, morbidity and case fatality related to atrial fibrillation in Scotland, 1986-1996," *European heart journal*, vol. 22, no. 8, p. 693, 2001.
34. S. Stewart, N. Murphy, A. Walker, A. McGuire, and J. McMurray, "Cost of an emerging epidemic: An economic analysis of atrial fibrillation in the UK," *British Medical Journal*, vol. 90, no. 3, p. 286, 2004.
35. G. Moe and J. Abildskov, "Atrial fibrillation as a self-sustaining arrhythmia independent of focal discharge.," *American heart journal*, vol. 58, no. 1, p. 59, 1959.
36. J. L. Cox, R. B. Schuessler, H. J. D'Agostino Jr, C. M. Stone, B. C. Chang, M. E. Cain, P. B. Corr, and J. P. Boineau, "The surgical treatment of atrial fibrillation. III. Development of a definitive surgical procedure," *The Journal of Thoracic and Cardiovascular Surgery*, vol. 101, no. 4, p. 569, 1991.
37. J. L. Cox, "The role of surgical intervention in the management of atrial fibrillation," *Texas Heart Institute Journal / From the Texas Heart Institute of St. Luke's Episcopal Hospital, Texas Children's Hospital*, vol. 31, pp. 257–265, 2004.
38. M. Haissaguerre, P. Jais, D. Shah, A. Takahashi, M. Hocini, G. Quiniou, S. Garrigue, A. Le Mouroux, P. Le Métayer, and J. Clémenty, "Spontaneous initiation of atrial fibrillation by ectopic beats originating in the pulmonary veins," *New England Journal of Medicine*, vol. 339, no. 10, pp. 659–666, 1998.
39. M. Haissaguerre, M. Hocini, P. Sanders, Y. Takahashi, M. Rotter, F. Sacher, T. Rostock, L. Hsu, A. Jonsson, M. O'Neill, *et al.*, "Localized sources maintaining atrial fibrillation organized by prior ablation," *Circulation*, vol. 113, no. 5, p. 616, 2006.
40. M. Haissaguerre, L. Gencel, B. Fischer, P. Métayer, F. Poquet, F. Marcus, and J. Clémenty, "Successful catheter ablation of atrial fibrillation," *Journal of Cardiovascular Electrophysiology*, vol. 5,

no. 12, pp. 1045–1052, 1994.

41. P. Jais, D. Shah, M. Haissaguerre, M. Hocini, S. Garrigue, and J. Clementy, "Atrial fibrillation: role of arrhythmogenic foci," *Journal of Interventional Cardiac Electrophysiology*, vol. 4, pp. 29–37, 2000.
42. P. Jais, M. Haissaguerre, D. Shah, S. Chouairi, L. Gencel, M. Hocini, and J. Clementy, "A focal source of atrial fibrillation treated by discrete radiofrequency ablation," *Circulation*, vol. 95, no. 3, p. 572, 1997.
43. C. Pappone, S. Rosanio, G. Oreto, M. Tocchi, F. Gugliotta, G. Vicedomini, A. Salvati, C. Dicandia, P. Mazzone, V. Santinelli, *et al.*, "Circumferential radiofrequency ablation of pulmonary vein ostia: A new anatomic approach for curing atrial fibrillation," *Circulation*, vol. 102, no. 21, p. 2619, 2000.
44. H. Estner, I. Deisenhofer, A. Luik, G. Ndrepepa, C. von Bary, B. Zrenner, and C. Schmitt, "Electrical isolation of pulmonary veins in patients with atrial fibrillation: reduction of fluoroscopy exposure and procedure duration by the use of a non-fluoroscopic navigation system (NavX (R))," *Europace*, vol. 8, no. 8, p. 583, 2006.
45. I. Deisenhofer, M. Schneider, M. Böhlen-Knauf, B. Zrenner, G. Ndrepepa, S. Schmieder, S. Weber, J. Schreieck, S. Weyerbrock, and C. Schmitt, "Circumferential mapping and electric isolation of pulmonary veins in patients with atrial fibrillation," *The American journal of cardiology*, vol. 91, no. 2, pp. 159–163, 2003.
46. S. Ernst, F. Ouyang, F. Löber, M. Antz, and K. Kuck, "Catheter-induced linear lesions in the left atrium in patients with atrial fibrillation: An electroanatomic study," *Journal of the American College of Cardiology*, vol. 42, no. 7, pp. 1271–1282, 2003.
47. R. Tilz, F. Ouyang, J. Chun, B. Schmidt, K. Satomi, T. Zerm, S. Ernst, B. Kokturk, I. Koster, and K. Kuck, "Ablation von paroxysmalem und persistierendem Vorhofflimmern mit der Doppel-Lasso-Technik," *Journal für Kardiologie*, vol. 14, p. 3, 2007.
48. H. Nathan and M. Eliakim, "The junction between the left atrium and the pulmonary veins: An anatomic study of human hearts," *Circulation*, vol. 34, no. 3, pp. 412–422, 1966.
49. M. Wijffels, C. Kirchhof, R. Dorland, and M. Allessie, "Atrial fibrillation begets atrial fibrillation: A study in awake chronically instrumented goats," *Circulation*, vol. 92, no. 7, p. 1954, 1995.
50. L. Yue, J. Feng, R. Gaspo, G. Li, Z. Wang, and S. Nattel, "Ionic remodeling underlying action potential changes in a canine model of atrial fibrillation," *Circulation research*, vol. 81, no. 4, p. 512, 1997.
51. M. Allessie, J. Ausma, and U. Schotten, "Electrical, contractile and structural remodeling during atrial fibrillation," *Cardiovascular research*, vol. 54, no. 2, p. 230, 2002.
52. D. Li, K. Shinagawa, L. Pang, T. Leung, S. Cardin, Z. Wang, and S. Nattel, "Effects of angiotensin-converting enzyme inhibition on the development of the atrial fibrillation substrate in dogs with ventricular tachypacing-induced congestive heart failure," *Circulation*, vol. 104, no. 21, p. 2608, 2001.
53. J. Eckstein, S. Verheule, N. de Groot, M. Allessie, and U. Schotten, "Mechanisms of perpetuation of atrial fibrillation in chronically dilated atria," *Progress in biophysics and molecular biology*, vol. 97, no. 2-3, pp. 435–451, 2008.
54. M. Spach, J. Heidlage, P. Dolber, and R. Barr, "Mechanism of origin of conduction disturbances in aging human atrial bundles: Experimental and model study," *Heart Rhythm*, vol. 4, no. 2, pp. 175–185, 2007.
55. S. Verheule, T. Sato, T. Everett IV, S. Engle, D. Otten, M. Rubart-von der Lohe, H. Nakajima, H. Nakajima, L. Field, and J. Olgin, "Increased vulnerability to atrial fibrillation in transgenic

mice with selective atrial fibrosis caused by overexpression of TGF-{beta} 1," *Circulation research*, vol. 94, no. 11, p. 1458, 2004.
56. H. Neuberger, U. Schotten, S. Verheule, S. Eijsbouts, Y. Blaauw, A. van Hunnik, and M. Allessie, "Development of a substrate of atrial fibrillation during chronic atrioventricular block in the goat," *Circulation*, vol. 111, no. 1, p. 30, 2005.
57. H. Neuberger, U. Schotten, Y. Blaauw, D. Vollmann, S. Eijsbouts, A. van Hunnik, and M. Allessie, "Chronic atrial dilation, electrical remodeling, and atrial fibrillation in the goat," *Journal of the American College of Cardiology*, vol. 47, no. 3, pp. 644–653, 2006.
58. K. Konings, C. Kirchhof, J. Smeets, H. Wellens, O. Penn, and M. Allessie, "High-density mapping of electrically induced atrial fibrillation in humans," *Circulation*, vol. 89, no. 4, p. 1665, 1994.
59. M. Bettoni and M. Zimmermann, "Autonomic tone variations before the onset of paroxysmal atrial fibrillation," *Circulation*, vol. 105, no. 23, p. 2753, 2002.
60. O. Sharifov, V. Fedorov, G. Beloshapko, A. Glukhov, A. Yushmanova, and L. Rosenshtraukh, "Roles of adrenergic and cholinergic stimulation in spontaneous atrial fibrillation in dogs," *Journal of the American College of Cardiology*, vol. 43, no. 3, p. 483, 2004.
61. E. Patterson, S. Po, B. Scherlag, and R. Lazzara, "Triggered firing in pulmonary veins initiated by in vitro autonomic nerve stimulation," *Heart Rhythm*, vol. 2, no. 6, pp. 624–631, 2005.
62. J. Zhou, B. J. Scherlag, J. Edwards, W. M. Jackman, R. Lazzara, and S. S. Po, "Gradients of atrial refractoriness and inducibility of atrial fibrillation due to stimulation of ganglionated plexi," *Journal of Cardiovascular Electrophysiology*, vol. 18, no. 1, pp. 83–90, 2006.
63. P. C. Gillette, M. M. Swindle, R. P. Thompson, and C. L. Case, "Transvenous cryoablation of the bundle of His," *Pacing and Clinical Electrophysiology : PACE*, vol. 14, pp. 504–510, 1991.
64. M. Borggrefe, T. Budde, A. Podczeck, and G. Breithardt, "High frequency alternating current ablation of an accessory pathway in humans," *Journal of the American College of Cardiology*, vol. 10, pp. 576–582, 1987.
65. C. Schmitt, I. Deisenhofer, and B. Zrenner, eds., *Catheter Ablation of Cardiac Arrhythmias: A Practical Approach*. Springer, 2006.
66. A. Luik, E. Ücer, M. Merkel, I. Deisenhofer, and C. Schmitt, "Katheterablation des Vorhofflimmerns - wo stehen wir 2008?," *Kardio up*, vol. 4, pp. 133–148, 2008.
67. F. H. Wittkampf, T. A. Simmers, R. N. Hauer, and E. O. Robles de Medina, "Myocardial temperature response during radiofrequency catheter ablation," *Pacing and Clinical Electrophysiology: PACE*, vol. 18, pp. 307–317, 1995.
68. R. Ventura, T. Rostock, H. U. Klemm, B. Lutomsky, C. Demir, C. Weiss, T. Meinertz, and S. Willems, "Catheter ablation of common-type atrial flutter guided by three-dimensional right atrial geometry reconstruction and catheter tracking using cutaneous patches: A randomized prospective study," *J Cardiovasc Electrophysiol*, vol. 15, pp. 1157–61, Oct 2004.
69. H. L. Estner, G. Hessling, A. Luik, T. Reents, A. Konietzko, E. Ücer, J. Wu, C. Kolb, B. Zrenner, and I. Deisenhofer, "Einsatz des Navigationssystems NavX bei der Ablationsbehandlung von Vorhofflimmern," *Herzschr Elektrophys*, vol. 18, p. 131?139, 2007.
70. A. Hodgkin and A. Huxley, "A quantitative description of membrane current and its application to conduction and excitation in nerve," *J. Physiol.*, vol. 177, pp. 500–544, 1952.
71. M. Courtemanche, R. J. Ramirez, and S. Nattel, "Ionic mechanisms underlying human atrial action potential properties: Insights from a mathematical model," *Am. J. Physiol.*, vol. 275, pp. H301–H321,

1998.

72. G. Seemann, *Modeling of electrophysiology and tension development in the human heart*. PhD thesis, Universitätsverlag Karlsruhe, 2005.
73. F. Jondral and A. Wiesler, *Wahrscheinlichkeitsrechnung und stochastische Prozesse: Grundlagen für Ingenieure und Naturwissenschaftler*. Wiesbaden: Teubner, 2007.
74. U. Kiencke and R. Eger, *Messtechnik: Systemtheorie für Elektrotechniker*. Springer Verlag, 2001.
75. H. Akkerboom, *Wirtschaftsstatistik im Bachelor: Grundlagen und Datenanalyse*. Wiesbaden: Betriebswirtschaftlicher Verlag Dr. Th. Gabler I GWV Fachverlage GmbH, Wiesbaden, 2008.
76. D. Massart, "Visual presentation of data by means of box plots," *LC* GC Europe*, vol. 18, 2005.
77. A. J. Izenman, *Modern multivariate statistical techniques: Regression, classification, and manifold learning*. Springer texts in statistics, New York: Springer, 2008.
78. C. E. Shannon, "A Mathematical Theory of Communication," *Bell System Technical Journal*, vol. 27, no. 3, pp. 379–423, 1948.
79. U. Kiencke, M. Schwarz, and T. Weickert, *Signalverarbeitung: Zeit-Frequenz-Analyse und Schätzverfahren*. München: Oldenbourg, 2008.
80. U. Kiencke and H. Jäkel, *Signale und Systeme*. München: Oldenbourg-Verl., 2008.
81. H. Lindner, H. Brauer, and C. Lehmann, *Taschenbuch der Elektrotechnik und Elektronik*. München: Fachbuchverl. Leipzig im Carl Hanser Verl., 8. aufl. ed., 2004.
82. V. K. Ingle and J. G. Proakis, *Digital Signal Processing Using MATLAB*. Thomson Learning, 2007.
83. K. D. Kammeyer and K. Kroschel, *Digitale Signalverarbeitung: Filterung und Spektralanalyse*. Studium, Wiesbaden: Vieweg + Teubner, 2009.
84. I. Daubechies, *Ten lectures on wavelets*. Regional conference series in applied mathematics ; 61, Philadelphia, Pa.: Society for Industrial and Applied Mathematics, 1992.
85. H. Nyquist, "Certain topics in telegraph transmission theory," *Proceedings of the IEEE*, vol. 90, pp. 280–305, 2002.
86. C. E. Shannon, "Communication in the presence of noise," *Proceedings of the IEEE*, vol. 86, pp. 447–457, 1998.
87. J. Bergh, F. Ekstedt, and M. Lindberg, *Wavelets mit Anwendungen in Signal- und Bildverarbeitung*. Berlin: Springer, 2007.
88. I. T. Jolliffe, *Principal component analysis*. Berlin: Springer, 2002.
89. W. Kessler, *Multivariate Datenanalyse für die Pharma-, Bio- und Prozessanalytik*. Weinheim: Wiley-VCH, 2007.
90. W. Martinez, *Exploratory Data Analysis with Matlab*. Boca Raton: CRC Press, 2005.
91. L. Breiman, J. Friedman, C. J. Stone, and R. A. Olshen, *Classification and Regression Trees*. Chapman & Hall/CRC, 1984.
92. W. Härdle and L. Simar, *Applied multivariate statistical analysis*. Springer Verlag, 2007.
93. S. R. Safavian and D. Landgrebe, "A survey of decision tree classifier methodology," *Systems, Man and Cybernetics, IEEE Transactions on*, vol. 21, pp. 660–674, 1991.
94. J. R. Quinlan, *C 4.5 Programs for Machine Learning*. Morgan Kaufmann Publishers, Inc., 1993.
95. J. Han and M. Kamber, "Data Mining: Concepts and Techniques," 2006.
96. J. R. Quinlan, "Induction of decision trees," *Machine learning*, vol. 1, pp. 81–106, 1986.
97. M. Mehta, R. Agrawal, and J. Rissanen, "SLIQ: A fast scalable classifier for data mining," *Advances in Database Technology ? EDBT '96*, pp. 18–32, 1996.

98. T. M. Mitchell, *Machine Learning*. McGraw-Hill Companies, Inc., 1999.

99. J. R. Quinlan, "Improved Use of Continuous Attributes in C4.5," *Journal of Artificial Intelligence Research*, vol. 4, pp. 77–90, 1996.

100. A. R. M. Martinez W. L., *Computational Statistics Handbook with MATLAB*. Chapman & Hall/CRC, 2002.

101. K. Nademanee, E. Lockwood, N. Oketani, and B. Gidney, "Catheter ablation of atrial fibrillation guided by complex fractionated atrial electrogram mapping of atrial fibrillation substrate," *J Cardiol*, vol. 55, pp. 1–12, Jan 2010.

102. K. Nademanee, J. McKenzie, E. Kosar, M. Schwab, B. Sunsaneewitayakul, T. Vasavakul, C. Khunnawat, and T. Ngarmukos, "A new approach for catheter ablation of atrial fibrillation: Mapping of the electrophysiologic substrate," *Journal of the American College of Cardiology*, vol. 43, no. 11, pp. 2044–2053, 2004.

103. R. J. Hunter, I. Diab, M. Tayebjee, L. Richmond, S. Sporton, M. J. Earley, and R. J. Schilling, "Characterization of Fractionated Atrial Electrograms Critical for Maintenance of Atrial Fibrillation: A Randomized, Controlled Trial of Ablation Strategies (The CFAE AF Trial)," *Circ Arrhythm Electrophysiol*, vol. 4, pp. 622–9, Oct 2011.

104. A. Khawaja, *Automatic ECG analysis using principal component analysis and wavelet transformation*. PhD thesis, Universität Karlsruhe (TH), 2007.

105. R. Jane, S. Olmos, P. Laguna, and P. Caminal, "Adaptive Hermite models for ECG data compression: performance and evaluation with automatic wave detection," in *Computers in Cardiology 1993, Proceedings.*, pp. 389–392, 1993.

106. M. Mneimneh, R. Povinelli, and M. Johnson, "Integrative technique for the determination of QT interval," in *Computers in Cardiology*, pp. 329–332, 2006.

107. D. Donoho, "De-noising by soft-thresholding," *Information Theory, IEEE Transactions on*, vol. 41, no. 3, pp. 613–627, 1995.

108. H. Lippert, *Lehrbuch Anatomie*. Urban & Fischer, 2003.

109. A. Bollmann, D. Husser, L. Mainardi, F. Lombardi, P. Langley, A. Murray, J. Rieta, J. Millet, S. Olsson, M. Stridh, *et al.*, "Analysis of surface electrocardiograms in atrial fibrillation: Techniques, research, and clinical applications," *Europace*, vol. 8, no. 11, p. 911, 2006.

110. J. Slocum, E. Byrom, L. Mccarthy, A. Sahakian, and S. Swiryn, "Computer detection of atrioventricular dissociation from surface electrocardiograms during wide QRS complex tachycardias," *Circulation*, vol. 72, pp. 1028–1036, 1985.

111. J. Rieta and F. Hornero, "Comparative study of methods for ventricular activity cancellation in atrial electrograms of atrial fibrillation," *Physiological Measurement*, vol. 28, no. 8, p. 925, 2007.

112. J. Rieta, V. Zarzoso, J. Millet-Roig, R. Garcia-Civera, and R. Ruiz-Granell, "Atrial Activity Extraction Based on Blind Source Separation as an Alternative to QRST Cancellation for Atrial Fibrillation Analysis," *Computers in Cardiology 2000*, pp. 69–72, 2000.

113. F. Castells, C. Mora, J. Millet, J. J. Rieta, C. Sánchez, and J. M. Sanchís, "Multidimensional ICA for the Separation of Atrial and Ventricular Activities from Single Lead ECGs in Paroxysmal Atrial Fibrillation Episodes," *Lecture Notes in Computer Science*, vol. 3195, p. 1229?1236, 2004.

114. J. Pan and W. Tompkins, "A real-time QRS detection algorithm," *IEEE Transactions on Biomedical Engineering*, pp. 230–236, 1985.

115. J. Rieta, F. Castells, C. Sánchez, V. Zarzoso, and J. Millet, "Atrial activity extraction for atrial fibrillation analysis using blind source separation," *IEEE Transactions on Biomedical Engineering*, vol. 51, no. 7, pp. 1176–1186, 2004.

116. R. Sameni, C. Jutten, and M. Shamsollahi, "What ICA provides for ECG processing: Application to noninvasive fetal ECG extraction," in *Proceedings of the International Symposium on Signal Processing and Information Technology (ISSPIT'06)*, pp. 656–661, 2006.

117. J. F. Kaiser, "On a simple algorithm to calculate the 'energy' of a signal," *Acoustics, Speech, and Signal Processing, 1990. ICASSP-90., 1990 International Conference on*, pp. 381–384, 1990.

118. I. N. Bronstein, K. A. Semendjajew, G. Musiol, and H. Mühlig, *Taschenbuch der Mathematik*. Harri Deutsch, Frankfurt am Main, 2005.

119. T. Everett, L. Kok, R. Vaughn, R. Moorman, and D. Haines, "Frequency domain algorithm for quantifying atrial fibrillation organization to increase defibrillation efficacy," *IEEE Transactions on Biomedical Engineering*, vol. 48, no. 9, pp. 969–978, 2001.

120. L. Faes, G. Nollo, M. Kirchner, E. Olivetti, F. Gaita, R. Riccardi, and R. Antolini, "Principal component analysis and cluster analysis for measuring the local organisation of human atrial fibrillation," *Medical and Biological Engineering and Computing*, vol. 39, no. 6, pp. 656–663, 2001.

121. A. Potamianos and P. Maragos, "A comparison of the energy operator and the Hilbert transform approach to signal and speech demodulation," *Signal Processing*, vol. 37, pp. 95–120, 1994.

122. L. Kaufman and P. J. Rousseeuw, *Finding Groups in Data An Introduction to Cluster Analysis*. New York: Wiley Interscience, 1990.

123. G. Botteron and J. Smith, "A technique for measurement of the extent of spatial organization of atrial activation during atrial fibrillation in the intact human heart," *IEEE Transactions on Biomedical Engineering*, vol. 42, no. 6, pp. 579–586, 1995.

124. J. Ng and J. Goldberger, "Understanding and interpreting dominant frequency analysis of AF electrograms," *Journal of cardiovascular electrophysiology*, vol. 18, no. 6, pp. 680–685, 2007.

125. J. Ng, A. Kadish, and J. Goldberger, "Technical considerations for dominant frequency analysis," *Journal of Cardiovascular Electrophysiology*, vol. 18, no. 7, pp. 757–764, 2007.

126. J. v. Rango, L. Adams, C. Stellbrink, L. Thieling, and W. Amceling, "Entwicklung eines Auswertesystems für die minimalinvasive Therapie von Vorhofflimmern," *Biomedizinische Technik*, vol. 46, pp. 178–179, 2001.

127. K. H. Kim and S. J. Kim, "A wavelet-based method for action potential detection from extracellular neural signal recording with low signal-to-noise ratio," *Biomedical Engineering, IEEE Transactions on*, vol. 50, pp. 999–1011, 2003.

128. B. Chandra and P. P. Varghese, "Fuzzifying Gini Index based decision trees," *Expert Systems with Applications*, vol. 36, pp. 8549–8559, 2009.

129. C. Z. Janikow, "Fuzzy decision trees: Issues and methods," *Systems, Man, and Cybernetics, Part B: Cybernetics, IEEE Transactions on*, vol. 28, pp. 1–14, 1998.

130. R. P. Brent, *Algorithms for minimization without derivatives*. Dover books on mathematics, Mineola, NY: Dover Publ., 2002.

131. C. Olaru and L. Wehenkel, "A complete fuzzy decision tree technique," *Fuzzy Sets Syst.*, vol. 138, pp. 221–254, 2003.

132. S. Varma and R. Simon, "Bias in error estimation when using cross-validation for model selection," *BMC Bioinformatics*, vol. 7, p. 91, 2006.

133. A. Erdogan, *Elektrochemische Potentiale während Hochfrequenz-Katheterablation von Herzrhythmusstörungen: In vitro und in vivo Experimente und erste klinische Erfahrungen*. PhD thesis, 2000.
134. V. Kremen, L. Lhotska, M. Macas, R. Cihak, V. Vancura, J. Kautzner, and D. Wichterle, "A new approach to automated assessment of fractionation of endocardial electrograms during atrial fibrillation," *Physiological Measurement*, vol. 29, pp. 1371–1381, 2008.
135. F. Kusumoto, *Understanding Intracardiac EGMs and ECGs*. Wiley-Blackwell, 2010.
136. E. Aliot, M. Haissaguerre, and W. Jackman, *Catheter Ablation of Atrial Fibrillation*. Blackwell Publishing, 2008.
137. S. Shpun, L. Gepstein, G. Hayam, and S. A. Ben-Haim, "Guidance of radiofrequency endocardial ablation with real-time three-dimensional magnetic navigation system," *Circulation*, vol. 96, pp. 2016–21, Sep 1997.
138. J. M. Kalman, A. P. Fitzpatrick, J. E. Olgin, M. C. Chin, R. J. Lee, M. M. Scheinman, and M. D. Lesh, "Biophysical characteristics of radiofrequency lesion formation in vivo: Dynamics of catheter tip-tissue contact evaluated by intracardiac echocardiography," *American Heart Journal*, vol. 133, pp. 8–18, 1997.
139. F. M. Weber, *Personalizing simulations of the human atria: Intracardiac measurements, tissue conductivities, and cellular electrophysiology*. PhD thesis, Karlsruhe, 2011.
140. *EnSite System Modell EE3000 v8.0*. St. Paul, MN, USA, 2008.
141. D. Scherr, D. Dalal, A. Cheema, S. Nazeran, I. Almasry, K. Bilchick, A. Cheng, C. A. Henrikson, D. Spragg, J. E. Marine, R. D. Berger, H. Calkins, and J. Dong, "Long- and Short-Term Temporal Stability of Complex Fractionated Atrial Electrograms in Human Left Atrium During Atrial Fibrillation," *Journal of Cardiovascular Electrophysiology*, vol. 20, no. 1, pp. 13–21, 2009.
142. Y. Takahashi, M. D. O'Neill, M. Hocini, P. Reant, A. Jonsson, P. Jais, P. Sanders, T. Rostock, M. Rotter, F. Sacher, S. Laffite, R. Roudaut, J. Clementy, and M. Haissaguerre, "Effects of stepwise ablation of chronic atrial fibrillation on atrial electrical and mechanical properties," 2007.
143. T. Rostock, M. Rotter, P. Sanders, Y. Takahashi, P. Jais, M. Hocini, L.-F. Hsu, F. Sacher, J. Clementy, and M. Haissaguerre, "High-density activation mapping of fractionated electrograms in the atria of patients with paroxysmal atrial fibrillation," *Heart Rhythm*, vol. 3, pp. 27–34, 2006.
144. M. Haissaguerre, M. Wright, M. Hocini, and P. Jais, "The substrate maintaining persistent atrial fibrillation," *Circulation: Arrhythmia and Electrophysiology*, vol. 1, no. 1, p. 2, 2008.
145. I. Deisenhofer, H. Estner, T. Reents, S. Fichtner, A. Bauer, J. Wu, C. Kolb, B. Zrenner, C. Schmitt, and G. Hessling, "Does electrogram guided substrate ablation add to the success of pulmonary vein isolation in patients with paroxysmal atrial fibrillation? A prospective, randomized study," *J Cardiovasc Electrophysiol*, vol. 20, pp. 514–21, May 2009.

List of Figures

2.1 The Heart ... 7
2.2 Conduction System ... 9
2.3 Action Potential ... 10
2.4 Standard ECG Leads ... 12
2.5 Electrocardiogram ... 12
2.6 Left and Right Atria ... 13
2.7 ECG and EGM during Sinus Rhythm ... 14
2.8 ECG and EGM during Atrial Flutter ... 15
2.9 ECG and EGM during Atrial Fibrillation ... 15
2.10 Influence of Trigger and Substrate on AF ... 16
2.11 Mechanisms of AF ... 18
2.12 Feedback-loops of AF ... 19
2.13 Catheter Examples ... 21
2.14 RF Catheter Ablation ... 21
2.15 CARTO & EnSite NavX™ Principles ... 23
2.16 Mapping System Anatomy ... 23
2.17 Hodgkin-Huxley Cell Model ... 24
2.18 Courtemanche-Ramirez-Nattel Cell Model ... 28

3.1 Boxplot Explanation ... 35
3.2 Boxplot and PDF of a Gaussian Distribution ... 35
3.3 Boxplot and PDF of χ^2- and Normal Distributed Data ... 36
3.4 Signal Transformation ... 40
3.5 Wavelet Examples ... 42
3.6 Block Diagram of a 1-level Wavelet Filterbank ... 43
3.7 Block Diagram of a 3-level Wavelet Filterbank ... 43
3.8 Basic Concept of PCA ... 44
3.9 Binary Decision Tree ... 46

4.1 Atrial Geometry ... 58
4.2 Comparison of Uni- and Bipolar Electrogram ... 58
4.3 CFAE Classes ... 60

4.4 Baseline Wander Removal ... 65
4.5 High Frequency Noise Removal ... 66

5.1 Coronary Sinus Signal with VFF ... 68
5.2 Ventricular Far Field ... 69
5.3 VFF Removal Block Diagram ... 70
5.4 Measured VFF ... 76
5.5 Synthetic VFF ... 76
5.6 Generating Test Signals for Evaluating VFF Removal Algorithm ... 77
5.7 Evaluating VFF Removal ... 78
5.8 VFF Removal Result ... 79
5.9 Evaluation of Synthetic VFF Cancellation ... 80
5.10 Evaluation of AFlut 1 VFF Cancellation ... 80
5.11 Evaluation of AFlut 2 VFF Cancellation ... 81
5.12 Evaluation of SR VFF Cancellation ... 82

6.1 NLEO of a Damped Sinus ... 87
6.2 NLEO of a Chirp Signal ... 88
6.3 NLEO of Superimposed Sinus Signals ... 90
6.4 NLEO Output Example ... 91
6.5 Gaussian Low-Pass ... 91
6.6 NLEO Segmentation Algorithm Block Diagram ... 92
6.7 Segmenting CFAE Effect of Post-Processing ... 93
6.8 Active and Inactive Segments of a CFAE ... 94
6.9 Active and Inactive Segments of an EGM ... 95

7.1 Atrial Signal Examples ... 98
7.2 CFAE Classes Examples ... 98
7.3 Contact/Non-contact Signal Examples ... 99
7.4 Amplitude Histogram of EGMs ... 99
7.5 Activity Ratio ... 101
7.6 Mean Length of Active Segments ... 101
7.7 Results NLEO-based Descriptors ... 102
7.8 Electrogram with Analytical Signal ... 103
7.9 Similarity of Active Segments ... 104
7.10 Mean Similarity of AS ... 104
7.11 CFAEmean ... 105
7.12 Dominant Frequency Algorithm Block Diagram ... 106
7.13 Envelope Detection of EGMs ... 107
7.14 AFlut and AF EGM with their PDS ... 109
7.15 Reshaping Active Segments ... 109
7.16 Example of Reshaped Active Segments ... 110
7.17 Periodicity Detection During AF ... 112
7.18 Periodicity Detection During SR ... 112

7.19 PDS of Contact and Non-contact EGM 113
7.20 Wavelet Decomposition of a CFAE 115
7.21 Wavelet-based Fractionation 116
7.22 Phase Space Regions 117
7.23 Phase Space Representation of Different CFAEs 118
7.24 Phase Space Sample Ratio 119

8.1 Fuzzy Decision Zone 122
8.2 Evaluating Fuzzy Zone Width 125
8.3 10×10 Cross Validation 126
8.4 Barplot of Used Descriptors 130
8.5 Boxplots of Descriptors Used by the Best FDT 133
8.5 (continued) 134
8.6 Fuzzy Decision Tree 135

9.1 Contact/Non-contact Electrograms 138
9.2 Tissue Model 139
9.3 Simulated Excitation Propagation 139
9.4 Catheter Orientation 140
9.5 Detecting Catheter Contact Block Diagram 141
9.6 Simulated Electrograms — Influence of Distance 143
9.7 Simulated Electrograms — Influence of Orientation 144
9.8 Influence of Filtering Electrograms 145
9.9 Influence of Filtering Simulated Electrograms 145
9.10 Boxplots of Descriptors Used by the Best Decision Tree 147
9.11 Decision Tree — Catheter-Endocardium Contact 149

10.1 EnSite NavX™ Anatomical Map 152
10.2 EnSite NavX™ Descriptor Map 153

11.1 CS Signal during Sinus Rhythm 159
11.2 Clustering CS Signals SR 160
11.3 CS Signal during Atrial Flutter 161
11.4 Clustering CS Signals AFlut 161
11.5 CS Signal during Atrial Fibrillation 162
11.6 Clustering CS Signals AF 163
11.7 PCA Cluster CS Signals AF 164

12.1 3D Maps CFAEmean and CFAE Classes 166
12.2 3D Maps NLEOenergy and AR 167

13.1 Boxplot and PDF CFAEmean Regions 171
13.2 3D Maps of Descriptors 172

A.1 CFAE Class Descriptors — F1 – F3 181

A.2 CFAE Class Descriptors — F4 – F15 182
A.3 CFAE Class Descriptors — F16 – F27 183
A.4 CFAE Class Descriptors — F28 – F35 184
A.5 Contact/Non-Contact Descriptors — $D_c1 - D_c6$ 185
A.6 Contact/Non-Contact Descriptors — $D_c7 - D_c18$ 186
A.7 Contact/Non-Contact Descriptors — $D_c19 - D_c22$ 187

B.1 Point-electrode Catheter — Position 1 189
B.2 Point-electrode Catheter — Position 2 190
B.3 Point-electrode Catheter — Position 3 190
B.4 Point-electrode Catheter — Position 4 191
B.5 Point-electrode Catheter — Position 5 191
B.6 Modeled Catheter — Position 1 192
B.7 Modeled Catheter — Position 2 192
B.8 Modeled Catheter — Position 3 193
B.9 Modeled Catheter — Position 5 193

List of Tables

2.1 CRN Currents ... 27
2.2 CRN Constants ... 27

4.1 Overview CFAE Database ... 61
4.2 Annotation of CFAEs ... 61
4.3 Overview of CFAEmean Map Database ... 62
4.4 Overview of Contact/Non-contact Database ... 63

5.1 VASR of Different Atrial Rhythms ... 69
5.2 Explained Variance of Eigenvalues ... 74
5.3 Select PCA Components by VASR ... 74

7.1 Results of Amplitude Descriptors ... 100
7.2 Results of NLEO-based Descriptors ... 102
7.3 Results of Characteristic Frequencies ... 108
7.4 Results of PDS-based Descriptors ... 114
7.5 Results of PCA-based Descriptors ... 114
7.6 Results of Phase Space-based Descriptors ... 119

8.1 Example Data from the UCI Machine Learning Database ... 127
8.2 Comparison of Different Decision Tree Algorithms ... 128
8.3 Descriptors Used for FDT ... 129
8.4 Results of Descriptors Used for FDT ... 131
8.5 Wrong Assignments per CFAE Class ... 134

9.1 Catheter Orientation ... 141
9.2 Results of Descriptors Used for Decision Tree ... 147

11.1 Number of Clusters ... 162

C

List of Publications and Supervised Theses

Journal Papers

1. F. M. Weber, **C. Schilling**, G. Seemann, A. Luik, C. Schmitt, C. Lorenz, and O. Dössel, "Wave direction and conduction velocity analysis from intracardiac electrograms — a single-shot technique," *IEEE Transactions on Biomedical Engineering*, vol. 57, pp. 2394–2401, 2010.

2. F. M. Weber, A. Luik, **C. Schilling**, G. Seemann, M. W. Krueger, C. Lorenz, C. Schmitt, and O. Dössel, "Conduction velocity restitution of the human atrium — an efficient measurement protocol for clinical electrophysiological studies," *IEEE Transactions on Biomedical Engineering*, vol. 58, pp. 2648-2655, 2011.

3. M. Burdumy, A. Luik, P. Neher, R. Hanna, M. W. Krueger, **C. Schilling**, H. Barschdorf, C. Lorenz, G. Seemann, C. Schmitt, O. Dössel, and F. M. Weber, "Comparing measured and simulated wave directions in the left atrium — a workflow for model personalization and validation," *Biomedical Engineering / Biomedizinische Technik*, (in press), 2011.

Conference Contributions

1. **C. Schilling**, A. Luik, C. Schmitt, and O. Dössel, "Analysis of intracardiac ECG measured in the coronary sinus," in *4th European Conference of the International Federation for Medical and Biological Engineering*, vol. 22, pp. 260–263, 2009.

2. **C. Schilling**, M. P. Nguyen, A. Luik, C. Schmitt, and O. Dössel, "Non-linear energy operator for the analysis of intracardial electrograms," in *IFMBE Pro-*

ceedings World Congress on Medical Physics and Biomedical Engineering, vol. 25/4, pp. 872–875, 2009.

3. **C. Schilling**, M. Aubreville, A. Luik, C. Schmitt, and O. Dössel, "PCA-based ventricular far field cancellation in intraatrial electrograms," in *Biomedizinische Technik / Biomedical Engineering*, vol. 55, pp. 49–52, 2010.

4. **C. Schilling**, A. Luik, C. Schmitt, and O. Dössel, "Visualization of CFAE descriptors on patient specific 3D-atria," in *Biomedizinische Technik / Biomedical Engineering (Proc. BMT 2011)*, vol. 56, 2011.

5. **C. Schilling**, A. Luik, C. Schmitt, and O. Dössel, "Descriptors for complex fractionated atrial electrograms: A comparison of three different approaches," in *Journal of Electrocardiology (Proc. ICE 2010)*, vol. 44, p. e31, 2011.

6. **C. Schilling**, A. Luik, M. W. Keller, C. Schmitt, and O. Dössel, "Characterizing Continuous Activity with High Fractionation during Atrial Fibrillation," accepted at *7th International Workshop on Biosignal Interpretation*, 2012.

7. M. Aubreville, **C. Schilling**, A. Luik, F. M. Weber, C. Schmitt, and O. Dössel, "Detection of periodicity in complex fractionated atrial electrograms (CFAEs)," in *IFMBE Proceedings World Congress on Medical Physics and Biomedical Engineering*, vol. 24/4, 2009.

8. M. Burdumy, F. M. Weber, A. Luik, R. Hanna, M. W. Krueger, **C. Schilling**, H. Barschdorf, C. Lorenz, G. Seemann, C. Schmitt, and O. Dössel, "Comparing measured and simulated incidence directions in the left atrium — A workflow for model personalization and validation," in *Biomedizinische Technik / Biomedical Engineering*, vol. 55, pp. 50–53, 2010.

9. O. Dössel, M. W. Krueger, F. M. Weber, **C. Schilling**, H. W. H. Schulze, G. Seemann, "A framework for personalization of computational models of the human atria," in *Engineering in Medicine and Biology Society, EMBC*, vol. 2011, pp. 4324–4328, 2011.

10. M. W. Keller, **C. Schilling**, A. Luik, C. Schmitt, and O. Dössel, "Descriptors for a classification of complex fractionated atrial electrograms as a guidance for catheter ablation of atrial fibrillation," in *Biomedizinische Technik / Biomedical Engineering*, vol. 55, pp. 100–103, 2010.

11. A. Luik, **C. Schilling**, O. Dössel, and C. Schmitt, "Einfluss der segmentalen Pulmonalvenenisolation auf die Defraktionierung bei Patienten mit persistierendem Vorhofflimmern", in *Deutsche Gesellschaft für Kardiologie 75. Jahrestagung Mannheim*, 2009.

12. A. Luik, **C. Schilling**, M. Merkel, O. Dössel, and C. Schmitt, "Effect of pulmonary vein isolation on the mean fractionation and the mean dominant frequency of the left atrium in patients with persistent atrial fibrillation," in *Heart Rhythm 30th Annual Scientific Sessions of the Heart Rhythm Society*, vol. 6, p. 153, 2009.

13. A. Luik, **C. Schilling**, M. Merkel, T. Riexinger, O. Dössel, and C. Schmitt, "Effect of pulmonary vein isolation on the defractionation of the left atrium in patients with persistent atrial fibrillation," in *Heart Rhythm 31st Annual Scientific Sessions of the Heart Rhythm Society*, vol. 7, p. 34, 2010.

14. A. Luik, **C. Schilling**, M. Merkel, K. Schmidt, O. Dössel, and C. Schmitt, "Impact of energy and CFAE classification in patients with persistent atrial fibrillation — analysis by a newly developed automatic algorithm (fuzzy decision tree)", in *Deutsche Gesellschaft für Kardiologie 78. Jahrestagung Mannheim*, 2012.

15. A. Luik, **C. Schilling**, M. Merkel, K. Schmidt, O. Dössel, and C. Schmitt, "Impact of energy and CFAE classification in patients with persistent atrial fibrillation — analysis by a newly developed automatic algorithm (fuzzy decision tree)," accepted at *Heart Rhythm 33rd Annual Scientific Sessions of the Heart Rhythm Society*, 2012.

16. M. P. Nguyen, **C. Schilling**, and O. Dössel, "A new approach for automated location of active segments in intracardiac electrograms," in *IFMBE Proceedings World Congress on Medical Physics and Biomedical Engineering*, vol. 25/4, pp. 763–766, 2009.

17. M. P. Nguyen, **C. Schilling**, and O. Dössel, "A new approach for frequency analysis of complex fractionated atrial electrograms," in *Engineering in Medicine and Biology Society, EMBC*, vol. 2009, pp. 368–371, 2009.

18. S. Ponto, **C. Schilling**, M. W. Krueger, F. M. Weber, S. Seemann, and O. Dössel, "Influence of endocardial catheter contact on properties of the atrial signal

and comparison with simulated electrograms," in *Biomedizinische Technik / Biomedical Engineering (Proc. BMT 2011)*, vol. 56, 2011.

19. F. M. Weber, **C. Schilling**, D. Straub, S. Gurm, G. Seemann, C. Lorenz, and O. Dössel, "Extracting clinically relevant circular mapping and coronary sinus catheter potentials from atrial simulations," in *Lecture Notes in Computer Science*, vol. 5528, pp. 30–38, 2009.

20. F. M. Weber, **C. Schilling**, D. Straub, G. Seemann, C. Lorenz, and O. Dössel, "Localizing ectopic foci in the pulmonary veins from intracardiac ECGs: A simulation study," in *IFMBE Proceedings World Congress on Medical Physics and Biomedical Engineering*, vol. 25/4, pp. 645–648, 2009.

21. F. M. Weber, G. Seemann, **C. Schilling**, M. W. Krueger, and O. Dössel, "Towards patient-specific simulations of atrial fibrillation," in *The Cardiac Physiome: Multi-scale and Multi-physics Mathematical Modelling Applied to the Heart*, 2009.

22. F. M. Weber, **C. Schilling**, A. Luik, M. W. Krueger, G. Seemann, C. Lorenz, C. Schmitt, and O. Dössel, "Quantitative determination of wave direction and conduction velocity in the human atrium from intracardiac electrograms," in *Journal of Electrocardiology (Proc. ICE 2010) (Young Investigators Award Finalist)*, vol. 44, p. e14, 2011.

Supervised Theses

1. Stefan Ponto, "Analysen zur Unterscheidung von Kathetersignalen mit und ohne Endokardkontakt", Diploma thesis, 2010
2. Matthias Keller, "Charakterisierung und Analyse von räumlich-zeitlichen Erregungsmustern bei Vorhofflimmern", Diploma thesis, 2010
3. Marc Aubreville, "Time-Frequency-Analysis and Blind Source Separation of Local Atrial Electrograms", Diploma thesis, 2009
4. Minh Phuong Nguyen, "Signal-Analysis of Complex Fractionated Atrial Electrograms (CFAE)", Diploma thesis, 2009
5. Tobias Heiss, "Multivariate Zeitreihenanalyse von Langzeit EKGs", Diploma thesis, 2008
6. Tobias Baas, "Dynamics of QT-RR-Relation", Diploma thesis, 2008
7. Maxim Moge, "Analyse der Morphologie der T-Welle", Diploma thesis, 2008
8. Anil Agarwal, "Spatial-temporal Analysis of Multichannel Electrocardiogram with special Focus on T-wave", Master's thesis, 2008
9. Sudhakar Tummala, "Spatial-temporal Analysis of Multichannel Electrocardiogram with special Focus on P-wave", Master's thesis, 2008
10. Kubilay Cokgüler, "Untersuchung der Auswirkung digitaler Filter auf intrakardial gemessene EKGs", Student project (Studienarbeit), 2011
11. Bastian Glauner, "Analyse von CFAEs und 3D-Visualisierung von Information auf dem Atrium", Student project (Studienarbeit), 2009
12. Lara Kanbar, "Patientspecific Visualization of color-coded Atria", Student project, 2010
13. Maria Tarat, "Spatio-temporal Analysis of Multichannel Electrocardiogram", Student project, 2008

Karlsruhe Transactions on Biomedical Engineering (ISSN 1864-5933)

Karlsruhe Institute of Technology / Institute of Biomedical Engineering (Ed.)

Die Bände sind unter www.ksp.kit.edu als PDF frei verfügbar oder als Druckausgabe bestellbar.

Band 2 Matthias Reumann
Computer assisted optimisation on non-pharmacological treatment of congestive heart failure and supraventricular arrhythmia. 2007
ISBN 978-3-86644-122-4

Band 3 Antoun Khawaja
Automatic ECG analysis using principal component analysis and wavelet transformation. 2007
ISBN 978-3-86644-132-3

Band 4 Dmytro Farina
Forward and inverse problems of electrocardiography: clinical investigations. 2008
ISBN 978-3-86644-219-1

Band 5 Jörn Thiele
Optische und mechanische Messungen von elektrophysiologischen Vorgängen im Myokardgewebe. 2008
ISBN 978-3-86644-240-5

Band 6 Raz Miri
Computer assisted optimization of cardiac resynchronization therapy. 2009
ISBN 978-3-86644-360-0

Band 7 Frank Kreuder
2D-3D-Registrierung mit Parameterentkopplung für die Patientenlagerung in der Strahlentherapie. 2009
ISBN 978-3-86644-376-1

Band 8 Daniel Unholtz
Optische Oberflächensignalmessung mit Mikrolinsen-Detektoren für die Kleintierbildgebung. 2009
ISBN 978-3-86644-423-2

Band 9 Yuan Jiang
Solving the inverse problem of electrocardiography in a realistic environment. 2010
ISBN 978-3-86644-486-7

Karlsruhe Transactions on Biomedical Engineering (ISSN 1864-5933)

Band 10 Sebastian Seitz
Magnetic Resonance Imaging on Patients with Implanted Cardiac Pacemakers. 2011
ISBN 978-3-86644-610-6

Band 11 Tobias Voigt
Quantitative MR Imaging of the Electric Properties and Local SAR based on Improved RF Transmit Field Mapping. 2011
ISBN 978-3-86644-598-7

Band 12 Frank Michael Weber
Personalizing Simulations of the Human Atria: Intracardiac Measurements, Tissue Conductivities, and Cellular Electrophysiology. 2011
ISBN 978-3-86644-646-5

Band 13 David Urs Josef Keller
Multiscale Modeling of the Ventricles: from Cellular Electrophysiology to Body Surface Electrocardiograms. 2011
ISBN 978-3-86644-714-1

Band 14 Oussama Jarrousse
Modified Mass-Spring System for Physically Based Deformation Modeling. 2012
ISBN 978-3-86644-742-4

Band 15 Julia Bohnert
Effects of Time-Varying Magnetic Fields in the Frequency Range 1 kHz to 100 kHz upon the Human Body: Numerical Studies and Stimulation Experiment. 2012
ISBN 978-3-86644-782-0

Band 16 Hanno Homann
SAR Prediction and SAR Management for Parallel Transmit MRI. 2012
ISBN 978-3-86644-800-1

Band 17 Christopher Schilling
Analysis of Atrial Electrograms. 2012
ISBN 978-3-86644-894-0